TWO SMALL FOOTPRINTS IN WET SAND

TWO SMALL FOOTPRINTS IN WET SAND

THE UPLIFTING TRUE STORY OF A MOTHER'S BRAVE QUEST TO SAVE HER DAUGHTER

ANNE-DAUPHINE JULLIAND

Translated by Adriana Hunter

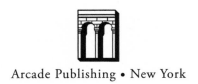

Arcade Publishing • New York

First Arcade Publishing paperback edition 2015

Originally published in France as *Deux petits pas sur le sable mouillé*

Arcade Publishing books may be purchased in bulk at special discounts for sales promotion, corporate gifts, fund-raising, or educational purposes. Special editions can also be created to specifications. For details, contact the Special Sales Department, Arcade Publishing, 307 West 36th Street, 11th Floor, New York, NY 10018 or arcade@skyhorsepublishing.com.

Arcade Publishing® is a registered trademark of Skyhorse Publishing, Inc.®, a Delaware corporation.

Visit our website at www.arcadepub.com.

10 9 8 7 6 5 4 3 2 1

Library of Congress Cataloging-in-Publication Data is available on file.

ISBN: 978-1-62872-444-8

Ebook ISBN: 978-1-62872-483-7

Printed in the United States of America

"Death's not a big deal. It's sad, but it's not a big deal."

GASPARD

THAT'S WHEN I FEEL THE WORDS RESONATE IN ME. THEY reach my heart and mind, infiltrating all of me: "If you knew ..."

Wednesday, March 1. An ordinary day, the end of a long, slow Paris winter. The waiting room, where we've been for twenty minutes already, is shoehorned between doorways to the neurology department at a children's hospital. We can see everyone going past from there. Every time a door opens, I stop breathing. I keep hoping—but also dreading—that I'll see the neurologist's face appear, and I'll know, at last. Since her call yesterday, time seems to be going on forever.

"We know what your daughter is suffering from. Come at three o'clock tomorrow, so we can explain it to you. Come with your husband, of course."

Since then we've been waiting.

Loïc is here, right next to me, pale, strained. He stands up, walks away, comes back, sits down, picks up a newspaper, puts it down again. He takes my hand and squeezes it with all his strength. My other hand strokes my rounded stomach—a gesture that's meant to be soothing for the little life that has been growing inside me for the last five months. An instinctive, protective gesture.

That's when I hear it. "If you knew ..." The phrase imprints itself deep in the heart of me. I'll never forget it. And I'll certainly never forget the way it made me feel: It was loaded with the suffering and confident calm of someone who knows—someone who knows everything. It single-handedly summarized the ordeal that would begin to shape our day-to-day lives in a few minutes' time.

The doctor arrives at last. She says hello, apologizes for being late and takes us into a small, isolated room at the end of a corridor. Two people follow us, one of them a specialist in metabolic disorders whom we have already met.

When we are introduced to the third person, my heart constricts: She's a psychologist. And then, with no warning, I'm overwhelmed by tears before I even know. Because all at once I've got it. "If you knew ..."

There isn't any thunder, and yet everything's roaring. The sentences reach me pared down to the essential points. "Your little girl ... rare genetic disorder ... metachromatic leukodystrophy ... degenerative effect ... very limited life expectancy ..."

No.

My brain refuses to understand, my mind rebels. They're not talking about my Thaïs. It's not true. I'm not here. It's not possible. I huddle against Loïc, my rampart.

While everything is scrambled inside my head, my mouth timidly formulates the words, "And for the baby we're expecting?"

"There's a one in four chance the baby will also be affected. A twenty-five percent chance ..."

The lightning bolt strikes. A terrifying black hole opens up under our feet. The future is reduced to nothing. Even so, in that terrible moment, our instinct for survival takes over for a few short but decisive seconds. No, we don't want an antenatal diagnosis. We want this baby. It represents life! A tiny glimmer of light on our grim black horizon.

The conversation continues, but without us. We no longer have the strength. We're somewhere else, nowhere. Now we have to get up and leave the room. It may not seem much, and yet it's one of the most difficult things to do. Because that move hurls us back into the present, into our lives where nothing will ever be the same again. It's symbolic: We have to pick ourselves up after the impact and carry on with our lives. A first step. A small step, but a step all the same.

We say good-bye outside the hospital, distraught, broken, shattered. Loïc is going back to work. Nothing had led us to anticipate a cataclysm like this.

I go home on autopilot. She's there, I've hardly stepped through the door before I see her, Thaïs.... . She's standing in the hallway with her great big smile, her pink cheeks, her cheeky expression, and her blond hair. There she is, happy, glowing, mischievous, confident. And today, Wednesday, March 1, is her birthday. She's two years old.

Thaïs is like any other little girl. Or at least she was until an hour ago. Until today the only distinctive thing about her was her birth date: February 29. A day that comes around just once every four years. With birthdays only in leap years. Loïc loves the fact. He announces happily that his daughter won't get old so quickly. There it is, her one peculiarity. That and a distinctive way of walking that's adorable but slightly hesitant. I noticed it at the end of the summer. I like looking at baby footprints in wet sand, and there, on a warm beach in Brittany, I realized that Thaïs walked in an unusual way. Her big toes turn outwards. She can walk, though, that's what matters. She might have some vague problem with flat feet, at the very most.

To set our minds at rest, we went to see an orthopedist in the fall. He didn't find anything wrong and advised us to wait a year to see whether things would straighten out by themselves. But a year is a long time for parents. And two opinions are better than one. We made an appointment at a children's hospital. They came to the exact same conclusion.

"There isn't any problem, at least not an orthopedic one," the doctor said. "But you should arrange to see a neurologist all the same. He might have an explanation."

We weren't worried; we knew there wasn't anything seriously wrong with Thaïs. It was clear to see.

October was drawing to a close. Our lives were brimming with insolent happiness. After Gaspard, who would soon be four, and Thaïs, we were expecting a third child in mid-July. By then, we would have moved into a bigger apartment. We were both fulfilled by our work, and we love each other. In other words, life was smiling on us . . . if it hadn't been for Thaïs's little foot which insisted on turning outwards as she walked. . . .

The neurologist couldn't see us before the end of the year. We were in no hurry, even though the caregiver and the principal at Thaïs's day care center think they've noticed tiny shaking movements in her hands. . . . and thought she didn't smile so much anymore. That was true, but we didn't find it alarming. Thaïs must have been aware of the still-invisible baby, she was feeling put out and unsettled by it. That must be the explanation. But it didn't stop her developing like every other little girl her age, singing, laughing, talking, playing, and marveling at the world.

When we met the neurologist, she confirmed all these facts, but went on to prescribe a series of tests. At the start of the new year, the MRI scan proved perfectly normal. Good news? No, not really, the doctors thought, because they still had to explain that gait problem. The diagnosis was looking gloomier. Thaïs underwent more tests, slightly more painful ones: blood samples, lumbar puncture, skin biopsy. We heard talk of metabolic disorders without really knowing what that meant and without any precise answers. For now.

Then Loïc and I were called in for blood tests. We went along meekly and confidently, light years away from suspecting what lay in store.

And yet, in a few days' time, our lives would be turned upside down.

"METACHROMATIC LEUKODYSTROPHY . . ." WHAT A BARBARIC name! Unpronounceable and unacceptable. Just like the illness it defines. Words that don't belong with my princess. There she is standing in the hallway, clapping and asking for her cake with its candles. My heart bursts. It's an unbearable sight. My daughter, who's so full of life, can't die. Not so soon. Not now. I hold in my tears for a few moments, long enough to give her a hug and settle her in front of her favorite cartoon. I close the door. She smiles at me.

My mom is waiting for me in the living room. I break down completely.

"It's worse than anything we imagined. Thaïs has something really serious. She's going to die. She's going to die."

Mom's crying. And she never cries.

I can't tell her more than that because I don't remember anything else. Before we left the hospital, the doctor, with some foresight, slipped into my hand a piece of paper with the name of the condition, "me-ta-chro-ma-tic leu-ko-dys-tro-phy." I separate out the syllables in an attempt to give them some sort of shape. To make the reality more concrete.

I have to start again three times before I can type the name into a search engine without any mistakes. I hit Enter. But I back down when it comes to clicking the links on the screen. I'm too frightened of finding the horror hiding behind them.

A message tells me I have an email. It's from Loïc. He's been braver than me. He's looked through sites on the condition and is sending me a toned down summary. Oh, I do love him! It is through his words that I assimilate what metachromatic leukodystrophy is. A nightmare. A combination of bad genes from Loïc and me. We are both healthy carriers of a genetic anomaly. And we both transmitted the defective gene to Thaïs. Her cells can't produce a specific enzyme, arylsulfatase A, which is responsible for processing a group of lipids, the sulfatides. Without this enzyme, these lipids accumulate in the cells and progressively destroy the myelin sheath, which surrounds nerve fibers and facilitates the transmission of nerve impulses. The condition is silent at first and then appears out of the blue. From that point on, it gradually paralyses the entire nervous system, starting with motor functions, speech, eyesight ... until it affects a vital function. The patient dies two to five years after the first effects are felt. There is currently no known treatment. Thaïs has the children's form of the condition, the most serious. She has no hope of recovery.

No hope. I can't breathe. "Two to five years after the illness started." But when did it start? Today? Last summer on the beach? Earlier still? When? I picture a huge egg timer with the sand streaming through it at top speed.

I reread the email, blinded by tears. I dissect each stage of the illness, right through to the end. I read that soon my baby, who's only just two, won't be able to walk, talk, see, hear, move, or understand. What will she have left then? "If you knew ..."

The phone never stops ringing. Daddy, my sisters, my in-laws, a few friends. I announce this cataclysm to each of them, repeating what I've managed to take on board. Each time, there's a cry of anguish, disbelief, and pain.

The bell rings in the neighboring school. Mom sets off courageously to pick up Gaspard. Thaïs's cartoon is coming to an end. A key turns in the lock; Loïc is home. In a few minutes, we'll all be together as we were at breakfast this morning. Like a normal family. Except …

We will have to share this news with the children. Gaspard comes in at full pelt, as usual. He describes in detail his hoop-rolling race in the schoolyard and, between two mouthfuls of his snack, announces triumphantly that he won again. What a contrast! For Loïc and me time has been left suspended since this afternoon, but life carries on at a hundred miles an hour for our little man.

I hug Gaspard, pulling him close to me. Loïc sits Thaïs on his knees. He speaks first and finds the right words:

"Today we found out why Thaïs walks the way she does. She has an illness that makes it difficult for her to move around. And to do other things too."

"I've know for a long time," Gaspard interrupts him. "I've known since I was little that Thaïs was ill. And I also know she'll soon be old."

We sit there speechless. To Gaspard, being old means dying. He's only ever seen old people "go." How can he understand?

"Is it my fault? Or daddy's? Or mommy's? And what about me, am I sick too? And you? And the little baby?"

He asks all these questions as if he had them ready beforehand.

Thaïs smiles a dazzling smile. She slips off Loïc's knee, takes three steps, falls over, and picks herself up, laughing. As if she were saying: "Now you know too. You get it." *She* already knows. She already knows so much more than we do.

We wish we never had to wake up, staying asleep forever, to avoid confronting the truth. How tempting! I envy Sleeping Beauty.... . It's been a difficult night, broken, tortured. Wide-eyed but grimly dark. The few short hours of sleep did allow me to forget, though. A bit. For a while. The previous day's images hammer inside my head: the doctors, their announcement, the emptiness. The nightmare becomes reality once more.

In the midst of the chaos in my mind, one glimmer of happiness—a sweet respite—magically hovering over the storm: Thaïs beaming as she blew out her two candles and giggling as she opened her presents. Gaspard singing "Happy Birthday" to his little sister at the top of his lungs. A standard family scene. But on that particular day, this moment of grace opened a window and let in the light.

Gaspard and Thaïs quickly went back to normal after we announced the bad news. Once over the initial emotion, they could think of only one thing: celebrating Thaïs's second birthday. Children have that ability to bounce back after tears. Because they don't project themselves into the future, they live fully in the present.

Gaspard and Thaïs's attitude reminds me of a lovely anecdote about people who are asked what they would do if they were told this was their last day. All the adults come up with great schemes, plan gargantuan meals, try to realize as many dreams as possible as quickly as they can. A little boy setting up his electric train set is asked the same question.

"If you knew you were going to die this evening, what sort of special thing would you do today?"

"Nothing, I'd carry on playing."

So, on this painful morning, when I'm not fully awake, still snuggled under my comforter, already succumbing to tears, I glimpse the solution: I will try to live in the present, informed by the past but never taking refuge in it, colored by the future but not projecting myself into it. In other words, do what children do. It's not just a rule to live by, it's a question of survival.

Loïc stretches beside me, then his features sag and his eyes redden. The reality has come back to him too. Brutally. I tell him what I've been thinking; he nods in silence and holds me in his arms as if sealing a pact. We will be united in this ordeal. It's our life. And we're going to live it.

A WEEK ALREADY. ONE HUNDRED SIXTY-EIGHT HOURS. TEN thousand eighty minutes. And as many minor victories. The battle begins again every morning when I wake and the thought needles through me: Thaïs is sick. And every day I cling to the simple actions of day-to-day life as if to a lifebelt. To stop myself going under. Wake Gaspard and Thaïs, without crying; give them breakfast and force myself to eat something; take Thaïs to her nanny and leave her there, without crying. Go to work. And actually work.

Every morning I'm tempted to abandon everything. Spend the whole day with Thaïs, clutching her close, covering her in kisses, and telling her I love her. What a wonderful schedule! But it isn't a life. It's a dream I'm keeping for later. For "up there." No, here, I have to carry on. For Loïc, for Gaspard, for our unborn baby. And for Thaïs, of course.

She's still the same little girl, engaging, unruly, cheerful, mischievous. And willful, very willful. So much the better. She'll be needing plenty of strength of character and fighting spirit to tackle the illness. She's not lacking in either at the moment. She never falls without picking herself up. She's not done amazing us yet.

In the space of a few days, we notice clear signs of her illness. Her hands shake. They already shook a little before, but we had chosen to ignore that. Now she has trouble putting the lid back on a felt-tip or bringing her spoon to her mouth. I want to help her. I even anticipate her every difficulty by doing things for her. She's infuriated. "No, Thaïs do it!" She wants to do everything, all on her own. I give in. On that and other things. I agree to all her wishes, comply with her every whim. I want her to get the most out of her life, with no constraints. I want her to be thoroughly happy. But the exact opposite is happening. I feel helpless. I don't know what to do to satisfy her now.

"Don't change anything," Loïc advises. "She can't understand why yesterday you would scold her if she did something wrong but today, without any explanation, you let her do it. She must think we've lost interest in what she does. Telling her about the illness hasn't actually changed anything for her, you know. In her little two-year-old's head there's no before and after March 1; life goes on like before. So we have to behave the same. We won't give up on her upbringing; we'll adapt it to the situation. It's important to keep a framework for her to be balanced and fulfilled. Thaïs is lost without the parameters we set."

It's true, he's right. I've already forgotten the anecdote of the little boy playing with his train set. . . .

"I want to have leukodystrophy too, so that everyone looks after me. But just a little bit of leukodystrophy, not too serious, not so mommy and daddy get worried." The psychologist listens attentively to Gaspard's thoughts. My little boy says this quite lightly, unwaveringly. These words, lobbed in halfway through a conversation, are very revealing about what Gaspard has experienced in the last few days. He's been doing this ever since we told him Thaïs was ill: saying what he's thinking, very openly. And he's grown tough on his sister. He puts obstacles in her way when she's walking; and when she stumbles, he doesn't help her but fervently encourages her to get over them or go around them, to cope with the situation on her own.

He confides his feelings to us with disconcerting candor. Gaspard is expressing himself, and that's a good thing. But we feel helpless when it comes to responding to him. We're finding it difficult enough managing our own pain. We have to reestablish some balance within the family, but right now we're reaching our limits as parents. Gaspard's questions are outside our competence. We can't be sufficiently objective to deal with them lucidly and serenely. So we turn to the informed, professional advice of a psychologist. She holds keys that aren't available to us.

She sees the three of us together in a comfortable room. Gaspard sits, facing her, with a blank sheet of paper and some felt-tips. At the psychologist's instructions, we describe the situation while Gaspard draws. Despite his apparent concentration, he doesn't miss a word of what we're saying. Our account goes right back to when Thaïs was born. Gaspard colors away more intensely.

"Sometimes," says the psychologist, intervening for the first time, "when a little sister comes into a family, the big brother isn't very pleased, because he's afraid people will lose interest in him. Then he imagines all sorts of terrible things happening to the baby. He might, for example, cast his own sort of magic spell on the baby to make her disappear. And if some time later the family finds out that the little sister isn't very well, that she's sick, then the big brother thinks that his bad spell has worked. He feels so sorry. He sees how sad his parents are. He feels guilty that his sister is ill, and responsible for how sad his family is. He's worried he won't be loved anymore. But that's not true, Gaspard, it's not your fault if Thaïs is sick. It's not because of anything you did. Look at me, Gaspard. It's not your fault; it's not because of anything you did."

Gaspard keeps his eyes lowered. He doesn't say a word. But every inch of that sheet of paper is colored. In places the paper is almost torn.

"And it's not your fault if you're not ill," the psychologist carries on, handing him a fresh sheet. "You're lucky to be well, you know. You have so many things to do in life—things that will make your parents proud and happy. And you don't need to have leukodystrophy for people to take care of you. But you have every right to say you want your own place in your family."

Gaspard stands up and comes to huddle between the two of us. Tears are streaming down my face like commuters familiar with the route. He's not yet four. His life is being built on these events. How can he stay balanced? Or believe in the future? How many boys his age know the world "leukodystrophy"? Childhood is all innocence and carefree fun. But, at such a young age, he is being confronted with adult concerns: sickness, suffering, and soon death. I want to spare him and protect him from all this. I want to reassure him once and for all of our absolute love. And yet again, in the eyes of my little treasure pressed close to me, I see a child's incredible strength. Gaspard is no longer afraid. He trusts us completely. He's been told, it's been explained to him, and he understands. He's accepted. We may have to repeat these things ten times, a hundred times. But each time, he will move forward slightly.

On the way out Gaspard seems happy.

"I like what the lady was talking about," he says with a smile. "She's interesting and kind. I'd like to talk to her again." And clutching his art in his hand, he adds: "I took the picture. I won't give this one to anyone. It's mine!"

Yes, my darling, it's yours. In that picture you expressed a part of yourself.

It's a revelation. So obvious. We pass a definitive milestone that day, almost without realizing it. We have an appointment in a different Paris hospital, with a professor who specializes in leukodystrophies. This meeting is important because, so far, our knowledge of the illness has been restricted to the snatches we remember from that first meeting and from information harvested on the internet. We have built up our strength a bit now, and we want to know more. We want to be prepared, to do battle as best we can.

Thaïs comes with us. The professor sees us with his collaborator and with the duty psychologist. We immediately feel we can trust them, even though we're both now so wary of men in white coats. Thaïs is relaxed too; she keeps smiling and joins the conversation in her own way.

The professor takes more than an hour telling us what he knows about this orphan disease. He answers our often blunt questions: We want to know when the various stages of degeneration will come, how and in what order, and when and how this leads to death. We want to know everything. Because when you know, you're not so

frightened. But it's impossible to answer all our questions as pre-
cisely as we hoped. There are still a great many unknowns in the
field—the illness is too rare. It affects just one child in several tens
of thousands. That's very few. And too many at the same time. In
the end, what the professor tells us backs up what we already know:
Thaïs will lose her faculties in a fairly short timescale. And science
can currently offer her no hope of a cure.

At the end of the visit, I get my princess dressed again on the
examination bed, with my back to everyone else: the doctors, Loïc,
and the psychologist. I am completely focused on her, her alone, and
I speak to her with all the spontaneity of a mother, a mother in pain:
"You heard everything the doctor said, my Thaïs. He's explained
that you won't be able to walk, talk, see, or move. It's very sad, it's
true. And we're very unhappy. But it will never get in the way of
us loving you, my darling, and doing everything to make your life
happy. I promise you that, my baby: You're going to have a lovely
life. Not a life like other little girls or like Gaspard, but a life you can
be proud of. And you'll never be short of love." Ours and the love of
so many other people.... .

From then on, everything is clear. So clear! We are going to move
the cursor that marks a life's timescale. Before we were told about
the illness, we had thousands of plans for Thaïs, thousands of hopes.
Enough for a whole lifetime. For a life that would end without us,
most likely at a respectable age. Now we have to move the cursor
forward, bring the finish line closer, shorten the timescale. And that
won't alter the most essential element in any existence: growing in
an atmosphere of love. Yes, Thaïs will learn love. Like Gaspard, like
other children, but in a shorter space of time. Thaïs's lifetime will be
more limited, yes, but it will be more dense. More intense.

The black and white world in our hearts is gradually taking on
some color again.

Amazing though it may seem, life carries on almost normally,
and we move house at the end of March. Everything carries on as

planned. We're happy in the new apartment, we now have more room, and we appreciate the extra space. Gaspard and Thaïs could have a bedroom each, but they would rather stay together. It's touching to see how well they get on together, accomplices supporting each other. It's touching and heartrending. . . . Shush! The present, nothing but the present . . .

We haven't moved far, only five Métro stations away. When we chose our new apartment, we didn't yet know that Thaïs was ill. We decided to keep Gaspard in the same school and Thaïs with her caregiver rather than finding arrangements for them near the new home. We were worried it would be disruptive for them. Changing halfway through the school year isn't easy. And, anyway, the school and the caregiver were near my office. It shouldn't be too difficult to organize.

What a mistake! The situation quickly proves impossible. All four of us catch the Métro together every morning. I get off with Thaïs before Loïc and Gaspard, who carry on another two stops. I climb the stairs to the surface carrying her in her stroller. Then I have a brisk fifteen-minute walk to the nanny's house. And another ten minutes back the other way to get to my office. Then the day's work begins. In the evening, I rush to pick up Thaïs, then, still rushing, we go to Gaspard's school, hoping we won't be late. Next, we hurry to the physiotherapist for Thaïs's motor skills treatment. After that the three of us head home in the Métro . . . or rather the four of us, because it's at this time of day that I'm particularly aware of my growing baby.

When I get home after more than an hour of this frantic pace, I'm just a shadow of myself, quite incapable of coping with the children who want a snack, a story, a game, a bath, a meal, a cuddle. All I want is to sink into the sofa and stay there. Loïc does everything he can to get home early, look after the children, make an effective contribution to this assault course, and offer me some relief. But he doesn't have enough time or energy. Our stamina takes quite a knocking.

One day I'm sitting flushed, breathless, and exhausted in the Métro, asking Gaspard to stop playing with the flip-down seats, and anxiously counting my contractions while Thaïs wails, when a man snaps at me, "There's no point having so many children if you can't cope with them." Absolutely zero compassion from this man who's clearly had his heart amputated! I'd like to hit him over the head, but I don't even have the strength to reply. I only manage not to break down. If he knew . . .

So when I get home, I pick up the phone to call mom, crying my heart out as I say, "I need help." I'm not asking for a single favor, I'm sending out an SOS. Help! I can't go on. Exhaustion is the ordeal within the ordeal. When you're overtired, you can't do anything constructive or see anything positive on the horizon. We don't need that. But it's still difficult to acknowledge that you're dependent on others, it takes a degree of humility to admit you've reached your limits. In this instance, though, I swallow my pride because doing so is vital. We'll never get anywhere if we carry on in isolation. It's the first time I ask for help. Not the last, oh no.

We soon realize we're not alone, far from it, and everything is sorted out quickly: A network of goodwill, from friends and family, is woven around us, like a parachute. It will never fail us, not in times of difficulty, nor in our everyday routine. I can't talk about it without a surge of emotion and gratitude for everyone, from near and far, who agreed to set sail into the storm with us and helped us stick to our course—and avoid capsizing.

From that day onwards, I never have to cope with Gaspard and Thaïs alone in the evening. There are lots of them—cousins, aunts, uncles, parents, friends—who answer the roll-call and take up their watch beside us. The days are less of a burden. I can catch my breath at last. Loïc too is less stressed.

Despite the comfort it affords us, it's still not always easy accepting help from other people. I learn not to say "thank you" every two minutes, to receive the kindness offered with total simplicity. I open the doors of our home, our daily lives, our intimacy as a family to other people. And I'm touched when I see the tact, respect, and efficiency in what they do. These are all forms of support, and they just keep coming. And still do.

Life becomes more organized. We have a taste of calm once more, a luxury we had forgotten. We start relaxing, managing to sleep again. Things aren't going too badly. . . . But the period of respite is brief because Thaïs's condition takes a sudden downturn: By early April she can no longer walk unaided and all her limbs shake. We find it very trying, but sadly, this is only the tip of the iceberg. The worst of it isn't something you can see, it's something we experience, painfully: Thaïs has frequent explosive screaming fits, particularly in the car. It's unbearable.

At first we put these scenes down to her feistiness: She must be rebelling against staying in her car seat. We try endless different tactics to stop these appalling tantrums: We get angry, pretend not to notice, console her, sing for her, laugh, cry. We change car seats four times. Nothing makes any difference; even the shortest trip turns into a nightmare. All of us, including Gaspard, dread going anywhere by car. And we eventually realize that something's not right. These outbursts are too violent, too frequent, too long, and too traumatic to be just tantrums. There's something inhuman about them.

We go back to the hospital that specializes in leukodystrophies for advice. There we discover an aspect of the illness that hasn't shown until now: pain. No, of course Thaïs isn't just making a scene. She's in agony, absolute agony. We learn a horrible new expression: neuropathic pain. This pain is associated with lesions on the nervous system; it can be searing and is resistant to classic forms of pain relief. It is often compared to a burning or stabbing sensation or to electric shocks. It's excruciating for parents to be told this. We have only one response: "Do something to make it stop!" The doctor prescribes a number of drugs to ease the suffering. Not the sort you would usually find in a household medicine cabinet. These are the first of a very, very long succession of tablets, syrups, pills, capsules, drops, etc., aimed at relieving our daughter's pain.

This impressive medication brings its own disappointments. We often need repeat prescriptions because we keep having to increase the dose as the screaming fits become more frequent. The pharmacists are getting to know us. But one day, I unexpectedly have to go to a different pharmacy. I hand over Thaïs's prescription as I glance at the beauty product displayed on the counter. The pharmacist reads it, looks up at me in astonishment and looks back at the prescription.

"Excuse me," she says eventually, "but who is this medication for?"

"My daughter."

"Your daughter? How old is she?"

"Two."

"Two? I'm afraid there's a problem here. They don't give this sort of medication to such a young child."

I wasn't expecting to be refused like this.

"I know it seems unusual," I try to explain, "but my daughter has a very serious illness. She has ..." and that's when I go blank! I just can't remember the name of this godforsaken condition. I concentrate, struggle to remember, try to describe it. Without success. The pharmacist is looking more and more skeptical. She turns to one of her coworkers who peers at me with the same suspicious look in her eye. I'm still desperately trying to remember the name, furious that my memory's letting me down in these particular circumstances. Still staring at me, they go to consult the pharmacy manager. As his eyes alight on the prescription, the words blurt out of my mouth: "metachromatic leukodystrophy." I've shouted it across the whole store.

"My daughter has metachromatic leukodystrophy," I carry on a little more quietly. "It's a degenerative genetic disorder ..."

The pharmacist looks at me compassionately, nodding his head. He knows.

"It's okay, you can give the medication to this lady, no problem." The woman who first served me comes back over.

"We're really very sorry," she says, handing the boxes over to me. "We never see prescriptions like that for such a young child. Next time we won't ask any questions."

As I head toward the door, clasping the bag to me like precious booty, she adds: "You hang in there, you and your little girl."

I SO MISS THAT LITTLE OUT-TURNED FOOT. IT WAS THAÏS'S distinguishing feature. I grew fond of it. It doesn't turn outwards anymore, because she can't walk now. Not at all. Not holding someone's hand, or leaning against the wall, or using a walker. Her legs have given up; it's too difficult. The brain had stopped sending them the right information. They fought valiantly, but eventually they let go. Thaïs will never leave her little footprints in wet sand again.

Even with the best will in the world, there's no fighting an enemy as stealthy as this illness. Thaïs has given in. Sometimes people talk about losing a battle but not the war. Sadly, I'm afraid we won't be winning any battles—or the war—against metachromatic leukodystrophy. It will have the last word.

Unless the battle isn't the one we think it is. What if the fight were actually going on in a different arena? True, Thaïs can't walk anymore, but has she actually lost anything because of that? She certainly doesn't look defeated. Quite the opposite. She's gathering her strength to concentrate on other fronts and gaining in strong will, patience, and lucidity. She uses our legs to get about, guiding us by pointing at where she wants to go and saying, "There, over there," in case we don't get it. Thaïs knows what she wants more than ever. And what she wants isn't necessarily what we want.

We want her to grow up like other children, develop like other children, live like other children. We want her to be like other children because we're afraid. Afraid of the unknown, of her differences, of the future. But *she* isn't afraid. That's the way most really young children are. It's why they can jump fearlessly from a table into their fathers' outstretched arms. They're not afraid, and they trust us. That's where Thaïs gets her strength—and her serenity. She's not worried about tomorrow, because she's not thinking about it. And because she trusts us: She knows we'll be here, whatever happens. She wants to carry on in her own sweet way ... even if that way is steep and she can no longer walk. That way is her whole life. She tackles it as it comes along, not comparing it to anyone else's. She feels its difficulties but also appreciates its good times—all the ordinary little things that we don't see because we're blinded by sorrow and fear.

No, the little foot I love so dearly will definitely never turn outward again. But that won't get in the way of Thaïs's happiness. And it won't stop us from loving her. When it comes down to it, that's all she asks.

A dull thud. Thaïs has just fallen over. Again. It happens more and more often because she has trouble sitting upright now. She is on the floor in the bedroom, in the middle of a construction game that was demolished by her fall. She's crying, and I go to help her. Gaspard is beside her, trying to sit her back up. I can see how upset he is but can't help reprimanding him, as I do every time Thaïs hurts herself when they're together. Once again I tell him that he must keep a closer eye on his little sister. I explain for the umpteenth time that she's sick, she's not as tough as he is. I take Thaïs in my arms to comfort her, and leave Gaspard on his own, crestfallen, in the middle of the room.

The sound of sobbing reaches me in the living room, so I go back into Gaspard's bedroom. He's on his bed, crying, with his head buried in his pillow. I've never seen him so desolate. It breaks my heart.

"Mommy, it's too difficult for me having a little sister like Thaïs. Not because it's Thaïs but because she's sick. My friends are lucky because their sisters aren't sick. I always have to be careful when I play with her. It's too hard for me. I'm not her daddy, I'm not her mommy, I'm not a grown-up. I'm just a kid. Kids don't look after other kids like that. It's the grown-ups who do that. I don't want to play with her anymore, because I'm too scared she'll hurt herself and I'll get into trouble. But it's not my fault if she falls over, it's because she has leukodystrophy."

I sit down next to him; he's knocked the breath out of me. He is so right. . . . I'd never thought of it. Or at least not like this. I have to recognize that I've lost all objectivity. My primary concern is Thaïs's wellbeing; I see situations only in relation to her because I'm so worried about her. And it's true, I project my concerns onto Gaspard by giving him responsibilities beyond his years. He's not even five years old. . . . My behavior means he can't be natural with Thaïs. He's afraid he won't be up to the job, won't be able to stop his sister from hurting herself, and will disappoint his parents and be scolded. Of course, a brother shouldn't be responsible for his little sister, whether or not she's sick. I'm sorry, Gaspard. You go back to being a little boy.

He's the one who comforts me. And finds the key: "I know what we're going to do, mommy. When I'm with Thaïs and something goes wrong, I'll shout 'Problem!' and you can come see what's going on. And you'll take care of Thaïs. Then I can just play with her. You know, mommy, I really like playing with my little sister—even if she is sick—because I love her with all my heart."

A KICK WAKES ME WITH A START. I FEEL AS IF I'VE ONLY JUST gone to sleep. I look at my watch: four in the morning. Not just a feeling, then . . .

The pedaling session starts again, even harder. My baby definitely doesn't feel like sleeping and has decided it wants me for company! I press my hands onto my stomach. I want my hands to communicate to this little creature bursting with energy, to communicate my love . . . and all the things I can't tell it.

Pregnancy is often described as a timeless period. Some women have a sense of completeness, achievement, being filled with the promise of a new life. The last few months have been very grueling for us. And anticipating this baby's arrival hasn't allayed our fears. Far from it. On March 1, it only took a few words to annihilate the present and mortgage our future. A one-in-four chance that this baby will also be sick. . . . A one-in-four chance that the nightmare will begin again. And it will be the same for any child of ours. We could look at things positively, saying that it means only a 25 percent risk . . . but that's 25 percent too much. Even one in a thousand is way too much for a parent.

I so envy mothers whose only concerns in those nine months are how much weight they're gaining and what name to choose for their little cherub! I envy them, and I resent them, given that I can't look at my stomach without shuddering in trepidation. They're so lucky! What a luxury their heedless expectation is! Better for them to stay that way; if we all had to bear in mind every possible disease and malformation, no one would have children at all.

All through March and April, I don't open my heart for a moment. I keep it closed so as not to dwell on my pregnancy. I try not to become attached to this tiny thing. Whatever happens, I mustn't think about the baby. Or I mustn't think about it finally being born. And us knowing. If I don't think about it, it won't hurt. Love makes us vulnerable, so I'm not letting myself love my baby; this makes the situation bearable.

Each time my maternal instinct resurfaces, I bury it as deep as I can. I want to hold back my love like I hold my breath. I'm torn in two by these conflicting emotions and contradictory feelings. Loïc is very aware that I'm trying to maintain some distance between the baby and myself. He can see my distress and feels it himself. He too is struggling to picture this life that's growing silently, even though, under normal circumstances, he's such an attentive, hands-on father: the sort who talks to his baby in his wife's womb, gets emotional at each scan, notices every kick, and impatiently counts down the days to the due date. We're saddened by our situation; we wish we could be thrilled and could prepare happily for our baby's arrival. So we reach a decision, one that may seem quite ordinary but is of paramount importance to us: We're going to ask whether the baby is a boy or a girl. And we're going to start calling it by its name from then on. By doing this, we hope to make this little creature more real, more a part of our lives.

"It's a girl." The technician pauses out of respect for our show of emotion. We're happy. Happy and sad at the same time. It's not easy picturing another little girl beside Thaïs. One's arriving, the other's leaving. . . .

We've chosen a name, and now we say it for the first time, in unison: Azylis. Azylis represents life, the future. And hope. In the silence of those sleepless nights when little feet drum against my stomach, I can't help feeling it's not just by chance that we're expecting her at this particular juncture in our lives. Azylis is here to rebuild our confidence. I cling to this idea and the hope that it offers. I feel I can hear her small voice whispering: "I'm here. I'm alive. Everything's fine."

I will be induced two weeks before my due date. We were given the opportunity to choose the date and decided that Azylis should arrive on June 29. A symbolic date for Loïc and me: We will have loved each other exactly seven years to the day. For better. And for worse.

Thursday June 29, three thirty in the afternoon. A breath. A cry. A life. Azylis is here, pink and adorable, screaming and alive. All at once, and with no warning, the dams break, love floods over me. I love you, my tiny little girl! And everything is forgotten: the sword of Damocles over your head, the horrors of the illness threatening you, the nights of anguish and hours of doubts, the concerns for the future, and my fear of love. I stop holding my breath. I can't hold my feelings back any longer. I love you!

Azylis makes time stand still in a moment of absolute happiness, as if the sun has suddenly, magically driven away the storm. There are no more signs of sorrow or rain. That is the miracle of life.

We cry hot, fat tears with the reassuring taste of emotion and joy. Yes, right now, we are truly happy.

I DON'T KNOW WHICH IS WORSE, BEING TOLD THE NEWS OR waiting to be told. Waiting requires disconcerting passivity: Everything is still possible, even the unthinkable. Waiting fuels doubts but doesn't give you the energy to throw yourself into the battle, even if you know in advance you won't win.

I watch Azylis sleeping in her Plexiglas crib, and I don't know what I'm seeing: hope or pain; a carefree life or the illness. I try to find the answer myself: Azylis looks more like Gaspard than Thaïs, so she should be spared. But genes don't follow that sort of logic. I take a different tack: If the nurse comes in before I've counted to ten, then Azylis isn't sick. But genes don't comply with superstition.

I can't get to sleep tonight, yet again. The joy of her birth is still with me, but it's darkening under an ominous shadow: fear.

Gaspard and Thaïs come this afternoon to meet their little sister. They both melt. Gaspard soon abandons the baby to focus completely on the Zorro costume we've given him to celebrate the birth. Thaïs, on the other hand, doesn't pay any attention to her fully-equipped new stove. She has eyes only for Azylis, stroking her and endlessly repeating, "Baby, I love you, baby." It's very touching watching these two little girls meeting for the first time.

Thaïs looks so big next to her sister. I look closely at her and feel quite worried: I left her barely twenty-four hours ago, and yet she seems to have changed. I notice how badly she shakes. Her head wobbles slightly. When she talks, the words jostle and collide in her mouth. She can't hold herself upright anymore but hunches her back. She's quite pale too. The illness is making its stealthy progress. My heart constricts in anguish.

I don't want to leave her again, ever. I'm afraid of not making the most of being with her, afraid I'll regret the time spent away from her. This wrenching feeling is truly trying and not something we can gauge adequately. It's everywhere: I want to spend more time with Gaspard, without neglecting Thaïs; I'd like to have quiet times with Loïc without feeling I'm abandoning my daughter. I need to split myself in two, in three, even in four to live my time with each of them to the fullest. I want everything to be possible. What a wonderful utopia ... the only safety net to save me from despair is still and always will be to live in the moment. Nothing more. *Carpe diem*? Not entirely.... There's nothing very carefree about our lives now.

Thaïs is getting frustrated. Her hair keeps falling over her eyes, and she can't push it back properly. The headband she's so devoted to must have fallen off somewhere between the car and the sidewalk. Gaspard is starting to climb up the walls in this confined space. Azylis is stirring; she's hungry. It's time to say goodbye. With a heavy heart, I kiss Gaspard and Thaïs, wishing them a good trip: Loïc is going to drive to Brittany and back, dropping them off with his parents. It feels like the other side of the world. We will join them in a few days, which feels like an eternity because I know what those days have in store for us: news that will send our lives toppling one of two ways. Definitively. For now I watch Loïc and the children walking away. Thaïs is leaving, and I miss her already.

Silence. A silence that roars and swells and bursts. A deafening silence. Worse than the shrillest scream. A silence as terrifying as the blackest void. It lasts a few brief seconds. A single breath. But a breath that takes everything away with it—all our hopes and all our joy.

The verdict is given: Azylis has the condition too. A window snaps shut on our dreams.

Tell me it's not true, that we're not sitting here in the consultant's office, looking like a pair of broken puppets. Tell me that! No. Sadly, no. The time for tears isn't over. Not at all, the ordeal is now twice as fierce. And our bodies are so worn, our hearts so tired, our minds so empty. The future, which we had pictured as something comforting and soft as an expanse of cotton, has turned into a field of thistles where everything prickles and tears. An endless field of thistles.

I'm shaking because Loïc is not showing any reaction. He's sitting on the sofa, staring blankly, his face ashen. Silent and distant.

When we were given the results, he just squeezed my hand a little harder. While my mind nosedived into an abyss of pain, Loïc was like a robot, talking to the doctors about what would happen next. As we left the consultation, he took Azylis's Moses basket without a word to my sister, who had been waiting in the corridor, and without a glance at his daughter. He didn't utter a single sound on the way home. A trip that seemed to go on forever.

Now he's sitting here, right next to me, but he seems so far away. And, for the first time, I'm really frightened. Up till now, we've always responded in unison. The *way* we thought about things was often different, but *what* we thought was the same. We experienced things together. We made our decisions jointly, although sometimes after a certain amount of discussion, but we have always been united. Loïc and I drew our strength from each other and knew that if we drifted apart, we should fear the worst. Which is why, right now, I wish he would howl and rant and rage. Anything, as long as he would react and say something. Then I'll stop shaking.

It's hovering there, gleaming, in the corner of his eye. And when it rolls down his cheek, it's like a fissure running through the wall that stood between us. A tear. A balm. A salvation. Loïc is snapping. We're saved. Our tears mingle together. Yes, we're crying over our future, but we won't go under, because we're together. Everything else seems far away now. Loïc's heart is next to mine. Right next to it.

It's night. The silence is suffocating, counterbalancing the turmoil inside me. I wake feeling stifled, with an imaginary vise tightening over my heart and head. A powerful painful sound rises up in my throat. A cry: "How? How are we going to cope? How can we get over a cataclysm like this? How can we live with all this suffering?"

Loïc takes me in his arms. He reminds me of an image that our loyal friend Father François used while preparing us for marriage. Loïc recalls his words: "Imagining a whole lifetime together is beyond our abilities. It's like trying to picture all the food we're going to consume in our lives. It makes you feel nauseous before you even start. Yes, it's enough to make you lose your appetite for the rest of your life. But if we settle for eating just what we want or need each day, without thinking about the next day's meals or the day after that, it feels imaginable. And yet, at the end of our lives, we really will have eaten that great mountain of food." I manage a smile hearing these words. They ring true. That's it: A whole life is made up of a succession of days.

The oft-repeated idea—sufficient unto the day is the evil thereof—has new resonance in the light of this reasoning. It offers me a safety valve. In order to survive, I will do things in stages. My view won't stretch over all the years to come, for fear of losing my mind. It will go only so far as the evening that closes each bustling day—each day with its difficulties but also its joys, however slight. Yes, we will live one day at a time. No more.

"Did you hear what I said? It's weird: I didn't ask why but how."

"Yes, you're right, it's strange. I haven't been wondering that either. But we could very legitimately ask why."

I think that in our innermost depths we know that this "why" could drive us crazy for the simple reason that there is no answer. We know the medical reasons, the wretched combination of bad genes. That's a valid explanation, but it's not an answer. Why this illness and this suffering? And why us? Why two children affected in our trio when the genetics imply a risk of one in four? But genetics don't let the laws of mathematics get in their way. They take their toll as they see fit. We have subconsciously faced the fact that we have no way of answering this "why," so we instinctively focus our attention on the next question: How?

From there we can start outlining solutions. And carry on living.

A BONE MARROW TRANSPLANT, THAT'S WHAT COULD SAVE Azylis. My ignorance of anatomy means I can't actually locate this much-discussed bone marrow. I identify it as the spinal cord but soon learn the facts by heart: Bone marrow is where blood cells are made; it produces white blood cells, red blood cells, and platelets. It is found inside bones, hence its name. A transplant involves replacing this marrow with some from a donor. New, healthy marrow that produces properly functioning blood cells. In Azylis's case, the transplant would mean she could make the enzyme she's missing, the famous arylsulfatase A, the cause of all our torment.

The professor mentioned this possible treatment during our first meeting last April. He anticipated using it on our then-unborn baby if the baby proved to have the condition, but not for Thaïs. It was already too late for Thaïs. Experience has shown that, with the infantile form of metachromatic leukodystrophy, there's no point in a transplant if it's given after the first symptoms have appeared. On the other hand, the earlier it is given, the better the chances of success. Today a handful of children with the condition have already benefited from bone marrow transplants. It appears to improve their lives, although not one of them is truly cured. But they were all older than Azylis at the time of treatment. Only by a few months, but a few months that could make all the difference. The diagnosis has never been made so soon after birth as it has with Azylis. Which is why there is so much room for hope.

The transplant needs to be made as swiftly as possible. Time is of the essence. The problem is almost mathematical. The transplant produces its full effect in the twelve to eighteen months following the actual treatment, and the first symptoms of infantile metachromatic leukodystrophy appear between the ages of one and two. We need to tackle the illness immediately and preempt it. We're in a terrible race against time.

There isn't a day to lose. The transplant doesn't happen just by clicking your fingers. Before the transplant, the patient's own bone marrow has to be destroyed using chemotherapy. This lasts, on average, a good week. Long enough to wipe out all the sick person's cells. Then the new marrow is injected into the patient. So much for the process itself; before we get to that we have to overcome a major barrier: finding bone marrow compatible with Azylis's.

Looking for a donor takes time, and time is infinitely precious to our daughter. The doctors immediately abandon the idea of a bone marrow transplant proper, thinking instead in terms of transplanting stem cells, which have the same properties as bone marrow cells. For us there are several advantages to stem cells: When a child is born, a sample of these cells is taken, frozen, and inventoried in dedicated tissue banks, so it is easily located and readily available.

The doctors are in the starting blocks to initiate their search. They need only one thing: our consent.

"Transplants are not without risks and consequences." We know this, but the doctor makes a point of reminding us. We have to make our decision with full knowledge of the facts. Of course the possibility of this treatment was mentioned during my pregnancy. We'd already weighed up the pros and cons and were prepared to launch into the adventure. It's easy picturing situations when they're abstract; it all gets more difficult when they become real. Azylis is here now. Truly here. So what to do?

Some patients die during the transplant process. You could say that doesn't change much in this case because, whatever happens, if we do nothing, Azylis will die in a few short years. But the two instances are different: on the one hand, because every day spent with her now matters; on the other, because if the transplant goes badly and Azylis dies, we might never forgive ourselves for making that choice and might feel directly responsible for her death. It's the fraught debate between acting and leaving things be. Between guilt and responsibility.

Another doctor reminds us that most patients who have had these transplants are unable to have children. This point may seem trifling, but we take it very seriously. You could look at this very pragmatically and say that, if Azylis doesn't have the transplant, she couldn't possibly have children because she won't survive to be old enough. But here too the situation deserves careful consideration; if we do something to try to cure her, we would actually be intervening in the whole process of the illness. And we don't know what sort of modifications this could trigger. If Azylis is cured, we would be happy with our choice. If she dies, we would bitterly regret our decision. But if she isn't completely cured . . . If she develops the illness up to a certain point and then stagnates for the rest of her days, even though she might not be in any danger ... she might resent us for intervening. She might hold us directly responsible for her infirmities and for her being sterile. Perhaps it's best not to intervene.

Of course we think it over, but in our hearts and our conscience, we believe it is our role as parents to try the transplant. Those of us who have children take action on their behalf every day ... we make decisions that affect them. And we do it with no sense of guilt, because we believe to our very depths that it's for their good.

We don't ask their opinion before feeding them, dressing them, or washing them. Making them better when they're sick ... or trying to. We are guided by our instincts as parents.

I remember some wonderful words from Professor Jean Bernard, an eminent oncologist. He would say you have to "add life to the days when you can't add days to the life." This quote inspires me in the commitment we're making for Azylis today. We're going to do everything to add some days to your life, my darling. Then we'll do everything to add some life to your days. Whatever happens.

WHAT A CRUEL DAY. THE MARQUEES ARE UP, THE FLOWERS arranged, the tables set. The sky promises to be clement on this beautiful Saturday in July. Thank goodness: Loïc's younger sister is getting married today. The house is buzzing like a beehive. All are getting dressed, getting ready, checking themselves in the mirror, putting on their finery. I unfold my dress, my head full of thoughts. I'm so out of place here. My colors are all faked, save the red of my swollen eyes. And the grey of my half-mast heart. I'm in mourning. In mourning for a future full of smiles. In mourning for my dreams. What an ugly irony of timing! I really don't feel like partying. My heart and body aren't up to it. Azylis is eight days old, and we've known for a scant forty-eight hours.

I spot Gaspard in the distance playing with his cousins in his pageboy outfit, which is already covered in dirty marks. He's not the same little boy as yesterday evening, the one I hugged with all my might to soothe his heartache. What a painful memory that is: When we told Gaspard and Thaïs ... when we told them that their baby sister was sick too, Gaspard fell apart. He'd transferred so much hope onto this baby. I read in his eyes the same sense of emptiness that haunts me.

"I can't be the only child in this family who gets to be a grown-up. I want to grow up with my sisters. It's not possible, mommy. Azylis can't be sick."

We tried to reassure and comfort him. In vain. No words can get the better of sorrow on that scale.

As for Thaïs, she was quite silent. Then she leaned toward the tiny baby and wrapped her in her little arms. She looked at her intently and murmured, "I love you, baby." That was it.

Gaspard was calm when he woke this morning. The night had driven away his pain.

"It's the party today. We're going to have cake and Coke and music. I want to go to bed the latest in the whole world."

I would have preferred to stay in bed and avoided going through with this day. The guests are starting to arrive. They look happy. People are kissing, chatting, laughing, clinking glasses. And I'm crying. But I am here. I'm not going to stalk about like a ghost or be a party-pooper. If I don't want our lives to turn into tides of tears, I need to learn to make the most of celebrations, recognize beautiful things, and appreciate the good times. And whatever my heart may think, today is party time. Which is why, as I put on my dress, I also put on a fitting smile. A bit forced perhaps. Who cares. I notice Loïc has reached the same decision: He's managed to overcome his sadness to be sincerely delighted for his dazzlingly happy sister. His strength gives me courage.

Azylis is so beautiful for her first outing into the world. Guests come to admire her one after another, each offering a wonderful compliment or a kind word. No one mentions her illness. By reading between the lines of a glistening eye, a slight pressure on my shoulder, or a more emphatic kiss on my cheek, I sense their unanimous compassion. I know that everyone dear to us is hurting today. Hurting *and* celebrating, like us. What better proof of their solidarity than their smiles. They know Loïc and I are using every ruse to look happy, so they're striving to support us in this effort. And for the first time that day I really smile. A smile full of tears, the good sort this time.

The cool of evening is closing in. Through my open bedroom window I can hear the sound of the festivities. Gaspard and his father are doing the party justice. They won't come in till dawn, happy and exhausted. Azylis is asleep, curled against my breast. Comfortably settled on my bed, I hum faraway tunes as I watch my pretty little girl. It feels good.

After that short family weekend, Azylis is hospitalized in Paris for two days of intensive testing. It's an opportunity to make a full assessment of her state of health; this will act as a reference point for the months to come. At this point the doctors notice that, even at this very young age, the illness is making its mark: The speed of her nervous conduction has already slowed imperceptibly. Azylis is also given an in-depth blood analysis to establish the precise composition of her blood; and, using that, every stem cell bank in the world will be quizzed in the hope of finding a bag of compatible blood somewhere.

While we are at the hospital, the professor gives us some disappointing news: The transplant can't happen in Paris. We're devastated; one of the Paris hospitals that usually carries out this sort of procedure is only five Métro stations from our apartment. Instead, for several months, we'll have to be expatriated more than a thousand kilometers away—in Marseille! Everything gets more complicated. Where will we live? What about Gaspard's schooling? And Loïc's job? How will Thaïs react in an unfamiliar environment, when she so needs to know where everything is? It's difficult to imagine making this trip in these circumstances. But we don't have any choice. Azylis's life depends on it.

The most urgent concern is to find somewhere to live in Marseille. The hospital offers us a room in the Parents' House, but it's not big enough for the whole family. And our absolute priority is to stay together. So we immediately send out an appeal. The grapevine works overtime, and it's not long before answers start coming in. It feels as if the solution falls from the sky: Chantal, a distant aunt I've never met, opens her home to us, and her heart. She doesn't know us but offers us her house in Marseille. A house big enough for all of us. And it's free until the end of September. More than we could have hoped for. Chantal doesn't even ask to meet us first; she instinctively trusts us. She is acting out of pure and simple generosity. I didn't know that still existed. Thank you!

There's more good news: The professor has already found a stem cell sample that matches the characteristics of Azylis's blood. It's in the United States. It's touching to think that at some point, somewhere in the United States, a mother gave some blood from her newborn's umbilical cord and that this blood could save our little girl today. Thank you, in English this time!

Everything is happening quickly now. We'll be moving any day, and Azylis is expected at the hospital in Marseille in early August. There she will have an operation to insert a central venous catheter, a kind of drip implanted deep under the skin. Then, on August 8, she will move into her quarters in the sterile room. For an indefinite period. Meanwhile, we don't want to waste a moment of our time as a family. We imprint ourselves with each other's presence. This precious time is cut short all too soon. Thaïs's condition takes a brutal turn for the worse.

THIS ISN'T JUST CHANCE, I'M SURE OF IT.

Thaïs held on until we came home from the hospital before she stopped talking. I think she even kept a reserve of tender words in the last days. She'd never said "I love you" so often. Then one morning, she stopped talking. Forever. The shock is appalling! We'd certainly noticed that, for some time now, she had to work for every word, but we couldn't have guessed that phase would end so soon.

Confronted with my mute little girl, I feel sad and lost. Having only recently turned two, she was just beginning to talk properly. Her last words still ring in the air, her stammered "daddy"'s and "mommy"'s. She'll never say them again. So how are we going to communicate? Being able to say what we want and like and think is so important. We need to talk if we are to express ourselves and understand each other—talking brings people together. I feel intimidated and pained by Thaïs's silence. But she doesn't. Here again, she accepts events completely naturally. She isn't thinking "never again" or "forever." She's living in the moment. And at the moment she can't talk. I feel like screaming for her, but she looks at us in silence, and that silence seems to say, "Trust me."

Do we have any choice but to follow her and give her the trust she's asking of us? We agree to follow blindly as she initiates a different form of communication. With the passing days, she teaches us to converse another way. She forces us into silence and invites us to hear something other than words. She modulates the sounds she produces, makes her expressions more intense and her gestures more precise. She develops a whole palette of smiles, movements, and thoughtful signs. She creates another language—her own. And thanks to this language, we can accept her silence into our lives. In order to understand Thaïs, we have to forget we have the gift of speech. Our every sense is on the alert: We watch her movements, decipher her sighs, and decode eye contact. Soon we're no longer even aware she's not talking. We feel as if we're hearing her, and we understand her perfectly. Thanks to her, we have a glimpse of how vast communication is beyond the realm of words.

I no longer miss her "I love you"s: I can't hear them, but I can sense them and feel them.

Sadly, Thaïs's decline is not restricted to the power of speech. During this already very trying month of July, I'm woken with a start one night by a premonition, and I go to her bedroom. I find her lying in bed burning up, her eyes rolled back and her body shaking. The emergency doctor diagnoses a state of severe dehydration and undernourishment. She's hospitalized immediately, and there the scales reveal the brutal truth: eighteen pounds! Thaïs now weighs only eighteen pounds!

In the last few weeks, she hasn't eaten much, very little in fact. Like not being able to talk, she's had a lot of trouble chewing and swallowing. We consulted a doctor who prescribed some high-protein creamy desserts. But that wasn't enough—to the point that her life is now threatened.

It's unthinkable: Thaïs was slowly leaving us, and we hadn't noticed how serious the situation was. It isn't negligence; we just didn't know. It was outside our scope as humans to grasp the scale of the disasters caused by this wretched illness. Even if you know what it's going to trigger, you can't integrate that into everyday life—particularly as Thaïs's condition isn't fixed; it keeps deteriorating, which means we have to adapt all the time.

This is the biggest problem with degenerative diseases: Nothing can be taken as a given. I think it's even harder to accept with respect to a child. The illness brought Thaïs to a halt right in the middle of the learning process. Walking, talking, potty-training, independence, all areas in which she had recently progressed. And they were all losing momentum already. I see her life as a grim bell-shaped curve: a gradual climb sharply interrupted and diving into a vertiginous fall. Yes, Thaïs's decline gives me vertigo. And this won't be the last of the pain … or the new discoveries. There it is echoing deep inside me again: "If you knew."

From now on, we need to be more vigilant and take seriously her every fever and her every change in behavior. For the time being, Thaïs needs to climb back up a nasty slope. She's so weak that she's struggling. She's given nourishment through a drip, and sometimes manages to eat a few mouthfuls. Each one is a victory. After a few days in intensive care, she is transferred to be near the medical team who usually take care of her. I can't go with her, because I'm getting ready for our imminent trip to Marseille. This separation is torture for me: I was so afraid of losing her, and now I'm worried about not being there for her when she needs me. This constant wrenching heartache. I ask my mother to stay by her side. She won't leave her for a moment, so I have nothing to worry about. Thaïs is well looked after in medical terms, mom is taking wonderful care of her, and Loïc spends every evening with her. I know she's in good hands. I just wish she were in mine.

WE ARRIVE IN MARSEILLE AS OTHERS MIGHT STEP INTO A boxing ring: with fear in their bellies and a furious determination to win. But unlike boxers who are masters of their discipline, we're heading into battle blind. There are so many unknowns for us. We've had no preparation for this sort of situation. Who has? The fight is hopelessly weighted against us. We feel as if we're facing an elite trained army. David was lucky he had only one Goliath to tackle. . . .

Amongst these hostile prospects, Chantal's house feels like a haven of peace. It's a little corner of paradise right in the middle of Marseille, with a pretty, shaded garden and cool, spacious rooms. The place emanates calm and tranquility. We instinctively know we'll feel right here, within these welcoming walls. This is where we'll come to draw new strength after days and nights of strain at the hospital.

Chantal isn't here, she left the keys with her daughter-in-law, Laurence, who shows us around the house. She greets us with the characteristic warmth of southerners.

"Welcome! You must treat this like your own home. And if you need anything at all, we're just next door."

The tone is set: We feel we're among family.

Gaspard is thrilled; he's always dreamed of living in a house. He's hardly out of the car before he's grabbed a big stick and gone off hunting for ants in the garden. We can hear him in the distance crying, "This is going to be great!" How wonderful to be so carefree . . .

My parents move in with us in Marseille. They were the ones who insisted on coming. When they first told us this plan, we had our reservations: We didn't want to implicate them too deeply in this risky adventure; we wanted to spare them. But their decision proved intransigent. And wise. They knew perfectly well that the two of us, Loïc and myself, couldn't look after our three children alone, for simple, logistical reasons: We don't have the gift of ubiquity! How could two of us manage school runs, meals, half days, weekends, as well as trips to and from the hospital? And all the unknown factors? It was unworkable, without an unrealistic choreography of tasks and a degree of energy we didn't have. So we accepted their offer very gratefully. In order to be sure we're never let down, they've arranged with my parents-in-law to work on a relay every two weeks, for as long as our exile in Marseille lasts.

My parents have taken the first watch. My father is particularly happy to be here: His southern blood instantly feels at home. He can't wait to introduce his grandchildren to the place where he was born. We each move into our quarters in the house. Once the mountain of suitcases has been unpacked, we savor a well-earned rest, particularly as tomorrow is likely to be very testing: Azylis is going into the hospital, and we're to be reunited with Thaïs, but not at home, unfortunately. She will be transferred to the same hospital as her sister. Two floors down.

This corridor has no secrets from me now. I've walked up and down it a hundred times. Every time the door to admissions opens, I run over: I'm waiting for Thaïs. Loïc went back to Paris early in the morning to accompany her on the journey. I can no longer control my impatience; I've already called him several times to know where they were. The last I heard, they had finally reached Marseille. They should be here any minute ... but don't the minutes go slowly when you're waiting! It's more than a week since I've seen Thaïs; I can't wait to see her. I hear the door to the corridor open again. I turn round. And there she is.

I smother her in my arms and cover her with kisses before having a proper look at her. Her cheeks are slightly fuller, although she's still very thin. She's pale and looks so tired. But she's got her lovely smile again. And that little spark of life is back deep in her eyes. Even though there's still a ways to go before she's really well again, I know she's on the right track. For now anyway.

Azylis stirs in her Moses basket. Soon she'll be in her own room too, two floors higher up. But right now she's visiting her big sister. Thaïs is really happy to see her again, and we're deeply touched by her joy. I believe there's a true solidarity between these two sick little girls. An instinctive complicity that goes far beyond mere blood ties. Gaspard is here too, standing proud between his sisters.

The setting is hardly auspicious for a reunion, but we don't notice the cramped room's impersonal walls or the nurses' intrusions. We're above all that. I wish time would stand still. Forever.

All good things come to an end. It's time for Thaïs's treatment. On top of the inevitable temperature and blood pressure checks that no hospital patient can escape, they need to change her nasal feeding tube. It's an unpleasant procedure for her and might be frightening for Gaspard, so we part again. Gaspard goes home; Azylis is moved to her new hospital room; and Thaïs gets her bearings in hers. Each going our separate ways.

From now on, the hospital will be our meeting place. Until Azylis goes into the sterile room, we can all meet where Thaïs is. We can even treat ourselves to a little escapade outside, in the hospital's playground. All five of us. Like a normal family.

ALL YOU CAN SEE ARE TWO BLACK EYES. TWO ASTONISHED EYES appearing from between an oversized cap and a disproportionately large mask. Azylis is bundled up in a sterile gown far too big for her. After a good clean-up with antiseptic, she's now dressed in the complete panoply compulsory for anyone crossing the threshold to UPIX (Unité Pediatrique d'Isolement X), the hospital's sterile unit. Dressed up like this, she looks smaller than ever. The unit isn't equipped with newborn-size outfits; they rarely have such young patients. Azylis is just five weeks old. . . . So we've made do with the means at our disposal. We've coped with worse; surely we could manage this: We rolled up the sleeves, knotted various bits, turned up the bottom. The end result isn't all that bad. Loïc appears in the same get-up, and I burst out laughing. It's the first time I've seen him in this outfit, which will soon become our uniform. I regret not having my camera with me! We're soon straight-faced again; the moment we've so dreaded has come. Loïc takes Azylis in his arms and carries her into the sterile room waiting for her. I go with them to the door of the unit.

When the door closes behind them, I realize I didn't kiss Azylis before she left. And it occurs to me that I won't be able to do so for several months ... kisses aren't allowed in the sterile unit. I already feel like an addict in withdrawal. The physical link connecting me to my baby is still very intense. I need to smell her, touch her, kiss her. The distance between us is so painful.

Access to UPIX is strictly regulated; you can't just walk in. Each patient can be accompanied by only one person at a time. No more. Also, visits are overseen. First, you have to ring the entry phone and show your credentials. A door opens onto a patio reserved for authorized visitors. From there they can see the patients—through glass of course, not directly. There's one window per room, and next to each window is a telephone for communicating with the patient inside.

Loïc will spend this first day with Azylis. I wait a while before appearing by the window. I peep my head up shyly. They're both in there already. Loïc is fussing around his daughter, checking all the fittings. Azylis is sleeping peacefully in her bed, now relieved of her cap and mask. Loïc has put her into adorable pink pajamas. She looks fine. But I'm not. I can't control my emotions. Now that she's actually in her sterile room, I have a glimpse of what's in store for her. And it terrifies me. My voice sounds strangulated through the intercom. I don't want to communicate my terror to Loïc, so I decide I should leave. I blow a kiss to my little girl from far away, so very far, too far. And I walk away.

I go downstairs to see Thaïs. She's sleeping too, and mom is watching over her. There's nothing more I can do at the hospital for now, so I go home to welcome Gaspard when he comes in from his walk. On my way home, I suddenly have to pull over in the shoulder lane. I cry till I have no tears left. I feel alone and empty, unbearably empty.

Get undressed. Put your clothes into the wardrobe. Take off your shoes. Put on the pants and gown. Slip on blue shoe covers. Disinfect your hands. Go through the changing room door. Wash your hands. Then disinfect them. Go through the second door. Walk along the corridor. Go into the airlock. Disinfect your hands again. Put a mask over your nose and a cap over your hair. Put on white shoes. Get into a sterile over-gown. No, the other way around, the over-gown first. Disinfect your hands and start again in the right order. Disinfect your hands again. Push the door to the room without touching the handle with your hands. Enter the laminar flow zone by pushing aside the curtain of vertical plastic slats—with your elbows, not your hands. And there, stop breathing. Or almost.

We repeat this ritual every time we visit Azylis. I hardly need to point out that it's better not to forget something outside—to prevent having to start all over again. Sadly, I have a terrible habit of leaving my car keys in my pocket in the changing room. How many times will Loïc come and ask me for them through the intercom when I'm comfortably settled in the room!

Despite these minor inconveniences, we willingly comply with the constraints of the procedure. These precautions are the price we have to pay to be in contact with our baby. And that's actually one of the advantages of coming to Marseille. Here children aren't isolated in a sterile bubble; they can live in a proper room. A small one, yes, but a room all the same, where they can have company. The room is cut into two separate areas by a curtain of plastic slats. The compartment where the sick person stays is equipped with a vertical laminar flow system: The ceiling comprises a stringent filter through which the air passes, and this decontaminated air sweeps vertically through the area. This is what ensures that the space remains sterile.

Where transplants are concerned, the enemy is microscopic. Every effort is made to flush out the tiniest bacterium, every last virus, the smallest microbe. Any contamination can have dramatic consequences, so the instructions are draconian: Every item introduced into the room must be sterile. The same goes for bottles, diapers, favorite blankets, toys, etc. Clothes are washed above boiling point and then delivered to the room in hermetically sealed plastic. Azylis's pretty little dresses haven't taken kindly to this treatment.... I quickly shelve any pride in her clothes and replace them with basic pajamas and bodysuits.

The germ wars would never be complete without a thorough daily cleaning routine. The maintenance team are seriously house-proud. They clean the room from top to bottom in record time. I take the opportunity to learn a few techniques that are as swift as they're effective. Always useful.

All the rooms in UPIX have the names of characters from the famous *Asterix the Gaul* cartoons. An irony of fate or a nod to the future, Azylis's room is called Obelix. It makes us laugh because Azylis is more the size of Dogmatix ... but she still has a legitimate place in Obelix's premises: She may not have his weight, but I'm sure she has the same strength as Asterix's invincible companion. And she fell into a cauldron as a baby too. In her own way.

The space dedicated to Azylis is especially small. The furniture has been kept to an absolute minimum: a cot, a TV, a table, and a phone. And an impressive panoply of medical equipment. There isn't room for an adult-sized bed under the laminar flow. But Loïc and I want to stay with our daughter day and night, so we're given a special armchair, which can be opened out and serves as a bed with only rudimentary claims to comfort. I'm thankful I'm only five feet three inches because I can shoehorn myself into the chair quite well without my feet sticking out. But it doesn't really matter how uncomfortable the furnishings are. Even with an excellent mattress and the softest sleeping bag, we wouldn't sleep well: perhaps because of the stress, certainly because of the confined atmosphere in there, and definitely because of the clothes. We're often too hot with all those layers on our bodies. And we'll never get used to sleeping wearing a mask.

We adopt the rhythm of three eight-hour shifts. Or nearly. Our days are carved into three blocks of time: one with Thaïs, another with Azylis, and the last at home to see something of Gaspard. The division is not very fair; the allocation is made according to how serious the situation is. Azylis takes a considerable share of our time because we alone are up to staying with her, and we don't want to leave her on her own. She's far too young. Thaïs also needs someone there all the time, but Mom can take turns with us. As for Gaspard, of course he needs attention, but he doesn't actually ask for much. He has a very busy schedule too! What with his expeditions in the garden, his walks around the old port, his trips to explore the city, and his afternoons on the beach—he never stops. One evening when I come home from the hospital exhausted, he throws his arms around me and says with a smile: "I'm so happy I'm having my vacation in Marseille. We're doing all kinds of new stuff. It was a good idea coming here." He hasn't yet realized we're not here just for the summer vacation. If he knew ...

I DIDN'T KNOW IT WOULD BE SO NERVE-WRACKING. IN ITSELF, it's not such a big deal, just a small hole in her abdomen, closed off with a "button." Direct access to her stomach so that it's easier to feed Thaïs. It's become vital to her. At first we opted for a nasal tube, and with that system Thaïs was getting the nourishment she needed, but it didn't suit her. The tube bothered her, and she tore it out as soon as the nurses' backs were turned. The doctors then mentioned a method that was more intrusive but far more effective: a gastrostomy. We tried to evade the issue until we were confronted with the bald fact: Thaïs can hardly swallow anymore. This obviously poses a problem with nutrition, but it's not just that. It's dangerous for her to be fed by mouth. With every mouthful, she risks a fatal wrong turn: The food might not follow the correct route and travel into the airways instead of the esophagus. So Thaïs will never be able to eat normally again. And that is what puts an end to our reservations.

The operation has gone well, and Thaïs is waking gradually. I lift the sheet; a small tube protrudes from her stomach, just above her navel. It's clean and neat, it doesn't seem to hurt her, it's practical and easy to access. Yes, there are lots of advantages, I know that. But I'm deeply affected by this procedure: I'll never be able to feed my daughter again. The frustration! It's so instinctive, the urge to feed your child. From now on, I have to program Thaïs's "meals" on a machine, determining when they should happen, how long they should go on, and how much she needs. I hate the thought of feeding her artificially on some far-from-appetizing-looking liquid. Never again will she experience the taste of good food, different flavors, something savory, something sweet. And she so loves her food. . . .

The nurse tears me away from my dark thoughts when she says, "I'm going to show you how to operate the force-feeder." Oh no, not that! How appalling! You can't talk about force-feeding when you're giving a little girl the nourishment she needs. She's not some goose in Périgord! The nurse used the term automatically; it's the recognized expression in the medical world. I have trouble containing my reaction but manage to ask her in a relatively calm voice not to use that word. She apologizes, very embarrassed, and corrects herself, "Is feeding system okay?" That's much better. From now on, Loïc and I scrupulously ensure that force-feeding remains exclusive to poultry. This isn't just quibbling about a word, it's to maintain Thaïs's dignity. In all circumstances.

As to outward appearances, nothing's happening. Azylis is sleeping peacefully in her cot, like all babies her age. She has good pink color, is breathing steadily, and has a regular pulse. Of course there are all these medical instruments around her, but aside from this equipment, everything seems normal. Only in terms of outward appearance . . . because on the inside, it's Hiroshima—the chemotherapy has just started. The principle of a bone marrow transplant can be summarized like this: Everything is razed to the ground and then built up again on new, healthier foundations. Right now, the bulldozers have been sent in. The timing is very precise. Azylis's entire blood cell production has to be wiped out in the space of a week, so the chemotherapy needs to be devastatingly effective and lightning fast. The dosage says it all. Azylis, at a tiny nine pounds, is given a dose equivalent to that meant for someone weighing 220 pounds! Obelix putting in another appearance . . .

We don't leave our pretty little Gaul alone for a moment. We scrutinize her every reaction, attentive to any suspect signs. But she seems to be coping with the shock. Every day, the doctors tell us how the chemo is going. They faithfully report back her counts of "polynuclear neutrophils," "erythrocytes," etc. These medical terms don't mean much to us, and the levels make little sense to us. Each time we have to decipher, understand, and then translate these very specific terms. Medicine struggles to succumb to accessibility. . . . The doctors explain in simpler terms that the blood cells are being rapidly depleted, so the treatment is working, and Azylis will soon reach the stage suitable for the transplant.

For now, we are doubly vigilant because, with her white blood cell count dropping, Azylis is stripped of immune defenses. She is entering a period of aplasia when any infection could be fatal. Right now, she has no defenses. Both literally and figuratively.

Azylis didn't want her bottle this morning. And it's the same again now, in the middle of the day; she's grimacing and crying with every mouthful. I don't understand what the matter is. We haven't changed anything, neither the teat nor the milk. Something's wrong. The doctor sheds some light on the problem: Azylis has buccal mucositis—in other words, the surfaces of her mouth and throat are ulcerated. It's one of the downsides of chemotherapy. So far, she's only lost her hair, which isn't very noticeable in a six-week-old baby who has bird fluff on her head.

Mucositis is a particularly painful side effect of the treatment—as unpleasant as having colonies of ulcers all over your throat. So Azylis is refusing to drink because it hurts. This is a problem because, whatever happens, she must keep up her strength. She really needs it. The solution is simple: She will be fed through a drip.

The installation process is easy: The drip is connected to the central catheter. This catheter, which was inserted under Azylis's skin before she was admitted to UPIX, is the compulsory route for every treatment she receives while in the sterile unit. It is through there that her medication is administered, her chemotherapy and, from now on, her food.

As of today, and for a period of more than two months, my baby won't drink a drop of milk. She will even lose the swallowing reflex. I feel so helpless: I can't feed either of my daughters.... That's hard for a mom to accept.

Why do things never happen the way we want them to? Thaïs was finally scheduled to be coming out of hospital. We were so looking forward to welcoming her to the house, and she couldn't wait to be home ... but, as luck would have it, today, the day she's been anticipating for over a month, she's not well, she's feverish and nauseous. The doctors are adamant: There's no question of her leaving the hospital in this condition.

This piece of bad news is the final blow for us. We're worn out; worn out from going backward and forward between one floor and the other, one room and the other, one daughter and the other; and worn out by constant concern for our daughters' state of health. We don't know where to find the energy to go further down this treacherous path. We wish we could have a moment's respite before Azylis's transplant starts.

Thaïs looks downcast. It's not so much because she feels sick, I know that: She's disappointed. Just like us, perhaps even more so. She's been here a long time, and she's grasped the fact that she now has to wait a few more days before she can leave. Patience isn't generally a characteristic of young children. And yet ... as she lies in bed sadly watching me unpacking her bags, she suddenly dries her tears, picks up a doll, and goes back to playing quietly, as if nothing has happened. She even gives a welcoming smile to the nurse who comes to take a blood sample. I sit down beside her and can't take my eyes off her, this little girl who never stops surprising me. I want to know what her secret is.

How does she endure all this with a smile? Where does she get the inner peace and strength to cope with so many trials? Of course, you could say she's just a child. You can believe that she's not aware of everything, she can't picture the future and quickly forgets unpleasant experiences, etc. Yes, of course. But it isn't just that, I can tell. Thaïs isn't tolerating her illness, she's living her life. She fights for the things she can change and accepts those she can't avoid. What wisdom! What a lesson! I can't help but admire her. And I'm not alone in that.

As the nurse goes out, she says gently, "See you later, Princess Courage. . . ."

MY HANDS ARE SHAKING ALMOST AS HARD AS MY HEART IS thumping. For the first and last time, Loïc and I are together in Azylis's room. UPIX's regulations allow this in exceptional circumstances, and today is certainly that. This August 25 isn't just another day: Azylis is going to have her transplant.

The bag of umbilical cord blood is here in front of us, more precious to us than gold. An oppressive atmosphere fills the already confined space in the room. We're finding it just a little harder to breathe behind our masks; we're feeling just a little hotter in our coveralls. The air has given way to a dense combination of nervous energy and excitement. I think this must be exactly what people call "palpable tension." A nurse runs through a list of final checks. Everything is perfect, the connections are ready, and Azylis is peaceful. The procedure can begin.

A bone marrow transplant is no more dramatic to watch than a blood transfusion. And transfusions don't impress me anymore; Azylis has already had several over the last week. I keep my eyes pinned on the drip system that carries on at a regular rhythm like a metronome. It will take nearly two hours to transfer the contents of the bag into Azylis's venous system. Two hours to change the course of things, of a life perhaps.

"Stop! Stop everything! It's not the right blood group." I leap up, gripped by uncontrollable panic, and scream across the room to make them stop the procedure right away. I've just read the letters AB+ on the bag of cord blood, but Azylis is blood group A+, I'm sure of it. They must have made a mistake! This is a nightmare! The doctor restrains me and reassures me: "Please, don't worry, there's no mistake. The two groups are mutually compatible. An A+ patient can quite happily be given an AB+ transfusion. It's even likely that, with time, Azylis will change her blood group and become AB+." I'm speechless with fear and shock. I would never have guessed that you could change blood groups. I have to admit that until I was confronted with the situation, I didn't know you could change your bone marrow either. . . .

I'm disconcerted now. Although I know she needs it, and it may even be vital to her, I can't get used to this intervention. Blood is one of those primordial things that we transmit to our children, but soon Azylis will be producing cells that are foreign to us. She will have a different blood heritage. No, our daughter's future is no longer in our hands. Nor in our blood either.

That's it, it's done, Azylis has had her transplant. She didn't notice a thing. We, though, are reeling from the storm of emotions. From this point on, we have no control over anything. By intervening in the hopes of curing our baby, we have unquestionably changed the course of things. But how? To what extent? What direction will her life take? So many unknowns freighted with hopes and fears.

We're not there yet, though. Before we start picturing potential improvements, we have to be sure the transplant takes well. The troops are in position; we now have to watch how they colonize Azylis's bone marrow. They need to be sufficiently effective to take over producing blood cells, generating their own red and white corpuscles, and platelets. But they mustn't be over-zealous. What can happen is that the transplant identifies the host's cells as foreign and attacks them. It's what's known as GVHD, graft versus host disease. It usually presents as skin eruptions.

I want a magnifying glass to discern the tiniest spot, the least trace of red. And God knows there are enough little outbreaks in newborns. Every day, there's some rash or patch or mark, something you wouldn't usually dwell on. I never worried about these harmless signs when Gaspard and Thaïs were babies. But I'm haunted by them now. Them and germs. Because Azylis is still in a state of aplasia.

Again, we increase our vigilance to avoid any sort of contamination. The antiseptic burns our hands, but we'd rather wash them twice than once. Every cough, every sneeze, every throat-clearing becomes suspect. To think that most mothers eagerly await their baby's first smiles, first teeth, and first utterances, and here am I, waiting impatiently for the first white corpuscles produced by Azylis's new marrow.

The next important stage is chimerism. Chimerism ... a wonderful-sounding word, almost poetic. It sounds like an invitation to take a trip through Greek mythology. But that's way off the mark! At UPIX, chimerism refers to the presence in one individual of cells from another. So, at regular intervals, Azylis's blood will be analyzed so that the number of cells from the transplant present in her bloodstream can be expressed as a percentage. It's one way of keeping up to date with the battle—like reports informing headquarters of the troops' progress. And the headquarters staff in room Obelix are waiting impatiently for the information. The first chimerism check is due in two weeks. A bit more patience.

ZABETH COMES THROUGH THE FRONT DOOR AND STOPS dumbstruck in the doorway: A singing human caterpillar is coiling gleefully around the living room, led by Gaspard brandishing a CD player, trophy-like, as it bellows out the decibels. Behind him is Loïc, following the tune in his powerful voice and squeezing Thaïs in his arms. I bring up the rear, struggling to keep up with the hectic rhythm of this improvised dance. We don't even see Loïc's sister come in. We're fully focused on our happiness: This afternoon, after an extra week in the hospital, Thaïs came home.

Zabeth puts down her bags and lets us drag her into the dance. She's come to spend a few days with us and was expecting to find us devastated and fraught. Yesterday, maybe. But not today. Today there's a party atmosphere. We've waited so long for this that we've even secretly feared it might never happen. But it has now; Thaïs is here with us. Our joy carries us along, and it carries us away in our dance. Gaspard has decorated the house, putting flowers in his sister's bedroom, leaving drawings on her bedside table, hiding candy under her pillow. I didn't tell him she couldn't eat candy. It wasn't the time.

Thaïs doesn't have a moment to catch her breath. She's hardly through the door before her brother grabs the stroller and shows her around the whole house, sharing with her his secret corners and his treasures and telling her about his life in Marseille. He takes her off into the garden, shows her his explorations and games, and points out the green budgerigars that nest in the park next door. He's introducing her to his new world, a world they're now going to share. At last!

Thaïs is completely dazed by so many novelties. It's an abrupt change for her when all she's known of Marseille was a hospital room. Her recovery is still shaky; we have instructions to be careful with her. That can be enforced tomorrow; today she and Gaspard are enjoying their reunion.

Zabeth, Loïc, and I also make the most of this happy interlude by celebrating: Ensconced in deck chairs, we sip a glass of chilled rosé wine. It's warm and pleasant, we can hear cicadas chirping and the muffled cries of supporters from the nearby cycling track. The sun is turning red as it goes down. Yes, this is definitely a good day.

It can't be helped. I can put flowers in a vase, scatter cuddly toys on the bed, and cover the walls with illustrations to my heart's content, but Thaïs's bedroom still looks like an adjunct to the hospital with the specialized bed, her stock of "food," the pouches for her meals, the compresses, bandaging, and tubing, and all the other equipment needed for her gastrostomy. Hospital life doesn't stop at the layout of her bedroom, it insinuates itself into our routine and sets its own rhythm. Thaïs is still going downhill. Her bouts of pain are becoming more frequent and intense, and the treatment to counter them is rising proportionately, to the point of becoming a real constraint. From dawn till dusk, not an hour goes by when we don't have to administer some medication or other form of care. Loïc and I are a little busier every day; we're simultaneously coping with the schedules of parents, nurses, and nurse's aides. I admit that it frightens me; I'm worried we're not cut out to cope. But it's the price we have to pay for the pleasure of watching Thaïs flourish at home.

During those weeks at the hospital when Thaïs was fighting to stay alive, the illness attacked her on other fronts. It cruelly tested her motivation. Thaïs can now hardly use her arms, she can't keep her head straight, and she can't sit up. But she still wants to sit, particularly at mealtimes; even though she's not eating, she always shows that she likes being at the table with us. We've tried our best to keep her upright in a highchair, but she found it very uncomfortable. To get around this problem, we've given her a specially molded chair, made to her measure. She's terribly proud of this new piece of equipment, especially as Gaspard says it looks like a princess's throne.

I'm finding it difficult to deal with the strain. September's looming, and we've now been living in Marseille for more than a month. A month of stress, fear, waiting, and exhaustion. A month of monitoring, constant attention, and endless trips between the house and the hospital. A month of quickly making the sign of the cross every day in the changing room at UPIX. A month of desperate struggle. A harrowing month, both physically and psychologically. And yet, our suffering is far from over. Will it ever be? My morale is failing, my convictions crumbling. I can't go on. I'd like to let myself go, be lighthearted again, and go back to a normal life. I wish I'd never heard the name of this damned illness. I wish I could rewind, change the settings, and start everything over. Only better . . .

Why doesn't that work? Why can't you press "reset" and erase the things that are wrong? I can't move forward anymore. I need a rock, a stick to lean on. Of course Loïc is here, always, irreplaceable. But he's too involved, he's right in the middle of the storm, buffeted and rattled like me. I beg Heaven to send us one of its lucky stars. Just one. If I knew … She will knock at our door on September 1, with no roll of drums or fanfare, and change our lives.

I've always believed in guardian angels. And in this topsy-turvy month, when we should be getting back to work or school, I find that our very own guardian angel is a Senegalese woman of forty who answers to the name of Thérèse.

Thérèse came into our lives as if by magic. Back in May, a cousin of Loïc's recommended her to us to look after the children. She spoke very highly of Thérèse's countless good qualities, both professional and personal. She thought Thérèse could be an invaluable help to our family, but we hesitated a long time before making up our minds. The situation was very different in May, and taking on a nanny didn't seem like a priority. At the time, we still thought we had the future ahead of us and time to tackle the developments in Thaïs's illness. We didn't know then that Azylis was also affected. We didn't know our lives would be blown apart.

Before meeting Thérèse, we anticipated carrying on with our arrangements without changing anything, keeping the children at school and the nursery, respectively. In the end, we allowed ourselves to be seduced by this opportunity, more for comfort than out of necessity. We made the decision barely three months ago. Soon it wasn't a luxury having Thérèse: She was absolutely indispensible.

In her work contract we wrote, "Take care of the children in the home." We might as well have put "be our cornerstone." Thérèse soon became a major part of our lives, the rock we used to keep our footing when everything was falling apart. She knew this would happen before we did. When I asked her whether she would mind cleaning and cooking for the children, she didn't take offence.

"I'm here to help keep the balance in your family," she replied generously. "So tell me what you need most, and it'll be my pleasure to do it."

When I called her in a panic to see whether she could come down to Marseille, she didn't have a moment's hesitation. She altered her plans, packed her bags, and came to join us without batting an eyelid.

Yes, Thérèse is an angel, a beautiful angel straight from heaven. She doesn't settle for just making our days easier, she makes them more beautiful. Simply by being who she is and doing what she does. Always with a smile. She has many more good points than Mary Poppins and that inexhaustible carpetbag! But Thérèse isn't a magician. So what's her secret? The love she invests in her every day-to-day action; she seasons food with it, sprinkles the washing with it, damps the ironing with it, covers the children in it, and perfumes the whole house with it. Her arrival marks a turning point in our story. With her, we discover a new way of perceiving our existence. She may not be aware of that, and will probably never know, because she isn't after honor or glory.

I have a strong conviction that our meeting Thérèse was not a chance occurrence. A kindly hand placed her in our path. And the children certainly need no persuading; they adopt her straightaway. Particularly Thaïs, who grants her complete trust. Instinctively. She must sense in Thérèse all the qualities of a good soul: the inimitable gentleness, the infallible patience, the constant good humor. And all those things that can't be described or written.

A little night music. The never ending litany of lullabies disrupting the nocturnal silence. Thaïs's nights follow the same unwavering pattern: Every evening, after the ritual of medication and prolonged goodnights, she falls asleep peacefully. But her rest always proves short-lived. Soon after midnight, forlorn chanting comes from her room. This long monotonous lament is barely audible but has the same effect on me as a piercing scream. It carries with it so much contained suffering and anguish. As if the ever-smiling, ever-positive Thaïs keeps her pain to herself all through the day, but by night the burden of it becomes too heavy to bear. Every evening, then, she calls out and asks for someone to keep her company and calm her fears that are amplified by darkness and silence. So we take turns to go to her, without fail.

With a flick of her eyes, she invites her visitor to sit down beside her, take her hand, and squeeze it gently. With an almost imperceptible gesture, she asks for her CD, a compilation of lullabies, always the same ones. During the day she likes listening to stories or songs. But not at night, never: Nighttime is the preserve of her music. With the very first notes, she relaxes. "Sleep, baby, sleep ..." The words transform the air into soft, enveloping, soothing cotton. Thaïs goes back to sleep, but if the hand loosens its grip or the music stops, she immediately reprises her plaintive litany. This can go on for several hours. We organize ourselves to spend the night by her side, drawing a comfortable armchair up to the bed and pressing a button so the machine plays the music on a loop. We snooze with her, until her breathing grows deeper and her hand heavier. Then, without switching off the lullaby, we can get up carefully and tiptoe out to savor some well-earned rest.

The first few evenings, I feel my strength abandoning me. I can't afford the luxury of repeated sleepless nights, the days are too demanding. I don't have the necessary resources to carry on at this pace for long. Once again, I've forgotten to take into account our faithful helpers. My parents and Loïc's take over these shifts, sparing us this responsibility. They take it in turns to spend a night with their granddaughter.

Her moaning is an efficient alarm system. At the first sound, the "night watchman" leaps up and goes to her, hoping she hasn't woken us. In vain. A parent's instincts can detect a child's call even through the deepest sleep. But we go straight back to sleep, knowing that our daughter is being pampered by one of her grandparents. These hours on watch are to produce a special bond between them. I thought they rather dreaded their watch and the prospect of a broken night.

Far from it: I realize they look forward to it with barely disguised impatience. In the secrecy of the night, she and they are getting to know each other better. They each relish these precious moments of complicity between a little girl and her grandparents. Because they know these times won't go on forever.

WE CAN BREATHE—THE TRANSPLANT SEEMS TO BE TAKING. Less than three weeks after the treatment, Azylis's white blood cell count is rising. They are being produced efficiently, and the risk of infection is gradually receding. Phew! The doctors seem pleasantly surprised by this relatively premature end to aplasia. It's an encouraging sign for further events; we're beginning to see the end of the tunnel. . . . And the first chimerism test reinforces our optimism: Ninety-one percent of cells present in our little girl's body are from the transplant. Azylis is a welcoming host!

These good results act on me like a soothing balm. They release the tension painfully locking my shoulders. They smooth the frown that forms a harsh furrow between my eyes. I let myself go. And I enjoy my baby with a carefree pleasure that has so far been prohibited.

Azylis is adorable. She's smiling, gurgling, flourishing. Almost all the side effects of chemotherapy have worn off. She no longer has any physical problems and isn't in any pain. She's doing well. Even though she still isn't eating, she seems in good shape. And literally in good shape ... well, okay, she's cheating a bit: Cortisone is giving her chubby hamster cheeks.

At UPIX there's always a psychologist available for parents who would like to see one. She regularly comes to visit me, and over the weeks we form a strong bond. I appreciate our conversations a little more each time and even catch myself looking forward to them. Her professional insight and the good sense in her ideas are useful to me in getting through this difficult period as best I can.

During one of our conversations, we discuss Azylis's wellbeing. We both agree that she displays a surprising *joie de vivre* given the circumstances. But if you really think about it, there's nothing surprising about this. The context isn't unusual for her, though it is for us. We're the ones who feel disorientated in this room, not her. This is her world; she knows little else because she's spent two-thirds of her existence between these walls. . . . All her bearings are in room Obelix. She's used to seeing us dressed in our masks, caps, coveralls, and shoe covers. She isn't frightened by the beeps from machines, the sound alerts of syringe pumps, or voices booming through the intercom. She's at home here. The nurses, touched by her, cosset and coddle her, and make the most of any opportunity to give her a little "spoiling," a hug that's typical of southern France. Azylis revels in the pleasure of having her mommy or daddy by her side the whole time—a privilege that plenty of children might envy her. Because that is a primordial need for a newborn: the parents' presence. So long as we're there, everything's fine.

"Mommy, when are we going home?"

Gaspard is sad. Now that the vacation is over, our time in Marseille is becoming difficult for him. He's realizing what he left behind in Paris, and missing it. He left his school, his home, his whole world. Of course he likes Marseille for the warm climate, being close to the beach, and the steady pace of life. But it isn't his world, he feels like a stranger here, and his life is getting a little tougher every day. He doesn't have any friends here; he feels too different. Yet he tries everything to adapt and be accepted.

"I spoke Marseillais in school today. I called one of the boys in my class *copaing*,[1] and after that he was quite nice to me."

Children can be merciless. . . . Despite the teacher's recommendations, her pupils don't seem very inclined to let Gaspard fit in. They think this little boy with a funny accent and two sick sisters is weird; some even call him a liar. It has to be said Gaspard set the tone from the start by being disconcertingly up-front.

As the only new boy in class, on the first day of school he introduced himself to his classmates like this: "My name is Gaspard. I live in Paris, not here. I came here because my sister has metachromatic leukodystrophy and she's going to die soon. And my other sister, who's just been born, is sick too. But my parents and the doctors here in Marseille are doing everything they can to make her better. So maybe she'll live. We don't know." The children stared at him, wide-eyed. They'd probably never heard anything like it.

The first recess revealed the gulf that had opened between him and them. In a matter of minutes, word had gone round the whole school; in a matter of minutes, Gaspard had become a fairground sideshow. Very few pupils dare go near him, many are afraid of being contaminated with this unfamiliar but clearly catastrophic illness. However hard Gaspard reassures them you can't catch it unless you're born with it, the kids keep their distance, whispering to each other about the new boy's bizarre life.

It's now nearly a month since Gaspard started school again, and the situation has hardly improved. He's wilting, surrounded by adults who are often tired and stressed. Thaïs's homecoming gave him back his smile for a while, but he soon realized he couldn't play much with his beloved sister anymore. Nowadays, the garden is his savior, his oasis. With his boundless energy, he always felt cramped in our

---

[1] The French word *copain* means buddy, and the southern accent typically puts a nasal "aing" sound at the end of words like this.

Paris apartment, but here he goes out into the garden every day when he gets home from school. He scatters crumbs from his snack to attract insects, tracks down crickets by following their chirping, or observes in minute detail some new beetle he hasn't seen before. He dreams up all sorts of adventures for himself, turning a thicket into a whole hostile jungle. But he's always alone in these imaginary odysseys. And I'm worried by his isolation.

When I come home from the hospital one evening, Gaspard runs out to meet me, shouting: "Mommy, mommy, I have a friend. A friend just for me."

He hardly lets me get out of the car, tugging at my sleeve and dragging me into the garden. There, in the shade of a cypress tree, I see a gleaming new cage. Inside I spy a ball of black, tan, and white fur huddled in a corner. Gaspard reaches his hand through the narrow doorway and gently catches the small animal.

"Mommy, I'd like you to meet Ticola. He's a guinea pig. Mamili gave him to me, but I chose him in the shop and gave him his name." His voice betrays tremendous pride and happiness. But then there's a note of concern as he adds: "Is it okay with you if we keep him? He's friendly. He hardly bites at all, and he gives me lots of cuddles. I've already told him about our family. Say yes, mommy, *please*."

I look at his sparkling eyes. My heart flips.

"Of course, Gaspard sweetheart! Do you know, when I was little I had a guinea pig the same color as yours."

I pick Ticola up and smile at his tufts of long hair, his small translucent ears and mischievous black eyes.

"Welcome to the family, Ticola. I'm happy you're Gaspard's friend. You take good care of him."

What a great idea Loïc's mother, Raphaëlle, had: giving Gaspard a pet. The two of them form an inseparable team. Gaspard tells Ticola what he's been doing each day, sharing his joys and confiding his sorrows. As soon as he's home, he gets Ticola and takes him everywhere with him. Sometimes I even see a little nose peeping out of Gaspard's pocket at mealtimes. . . .

Thaïs is also delighted with the newcomer. She likes stroking him and giggles with pleasure when he tickles her hand. She seems happy. As for us, we're relieved: Ticola makes Gaspard's life more complete; he's come and filled a gap that Thaïs was struggling to occupy; he's taken her place as a playmate. Gaspard doesn't expect so much from his sister now. He still spends happy times with her, but he no longer complains because they can't play together properly. As a matter of fact, it's the other way around—he includes Thaïs as their accomplice. He tells her in detail everything he does with his friend Ticola. He explains to her how he feeds him, looks after him, takes him on walks, and rocks him to sleep. In fact, he watches over that guinea pig the way we watch over Thaïs. One day, he actually looks at me with a worried frown and asks, "Mommy, are you sure Ticola doesn't have leukodystrophy?"

WARNING: THE INVADERS ARE BEATING A RETREAT! THE defenses are getting organized in Azylis's resident army and halting the alien troops' progress. The chimerism test indicates a worrying inventory of figures: Thirty days after hostilities began, the transplant cells are backing off.

No one's waving a white flag, and there are no signs of surrender, but the doctors are concerned by this tendency. The percentage of foreign cells should keep growing. The battle plan needs changing immediately to try to reverse the process. To do this, the doctors have to become skilled strategists. They're going to induce a programmed and controlled graft versus host (GVH) effect. The technique consists of encouraging Azylis's cells to attack the transplant in order to stimulate it and elicit a defensive reaction—rather like a mouse provoking an elephant. Then the revitalized transplant cells shouldn't have any trouble seeing off Azylis's own cells that have been weakened by chemotherapy. Once the field is clear, the transplant can carry on with its colonization.

This sort of guerilla warfare requires true mastery; the transplant mustn't get carried away and bombard our baby's cells too violently.

The attack needs to be proportional to the anticipated result. Described like that, it sounds like some sort of board game. Except there's nothing playful about this at all.

The medical team are used to frequent reversals in situations involving transplants. But we're not. It was all going so well till now.... We had everything to hope for. We were wrong to let ourselves be lulled by the good news. We lowered our guard, and now we're not ready to deal with the hard knocks. Last week, we started hearing talk about Azylis's leaving the hospital, although we didn't dare really believe it. Now everything hangs in the balance again. Our hopes have just gone up in smoke.

Our life is nothing but a succession of waiting games, U-turns, and unpleasant surprises. We spend our time shuttling backward and forward between joy and disappointment. I'm done with finding ways to stay positive, adapt, shelve plans, and start over. I want to go home and get back to our normal life, because back in Paris, although our existence still has exceptional parameters, we have a sense of everyday normality. This place is just a digression.

"Right, come on," Loïc says, picking himself up again. "We're not going to give in. We made a choice when Azylis was born; we committed ourselves to fighting alongside her against this illness. That's our only goal right now. Of course we want to be home. But that's incidental. What matters at the moment is that everything goes well for Azylis. And this whole episode becomes just a bad memory. Only then can we start thinking about leaving."

I sign the pact once again. Anyway, I don't have a choice, do I?

The time has come to do the counts. It's two weeks now since the GVH was set in motion. From the outside, we haven't noticed any changes. Azylis is still well; she's still smiling and babbling. Yet again, there's nothing to betray the battle being waged on the inside. Appearances certainly are deceptive.... We're waiting impatiently for the results. I'm with Azylis, and Loïc is keeping me company on the other side of the window.

The doctor arrives with a triumphant expression. The GVH is working as everyone hoped it would. The transplant cells are picking themselves up and multiplying at an exponential rate. Azylis isn't displaying any signs of complications. What a relief.

Sometimes good news comes in twos. . . . The doctor doesn't stop there. He tells us that the last set of tests are very encouraging in other ways, and the new bone marrow is doing its work: Azylis is back up to a normal platelet count, so she's no longer dependent on transfusions. There are also good levels of white corpuscles, which are responsible for immune defense, making her completely autonomous in this area too. She still needs to develop lymphocytes and red corpuscles, but everything seems well underway. So she's to be transferred without delay to a different hospital department: the "protected area."

Can someone pinch me, please! Did I hear that right? Is Azylis really going to leave her sterile room? What, *now*? Well, almost, as soon as everything's ready for her. What incredible news! We're over the moon. The protected area is something of an intermediary between the sterile room and home. The degree of isolation and sterilization isn't as strict as in UPIX. Of course, we still have to wear masks and keep to our hand-washing routines, but we won't have to go through that ritual of gowning and degowning.

I have one burning question: "Will we be able to kiss her?"

No, not yet, it's too soon.

But, deep down, I can tell the time is drawing near. We're taking a big step toward the doors to the outside world.

P AUSE. WE'VE PRESSED THE PAUSE BUTTON TODAY, JUST LONG enough to be alone together as a couple. We've entrusted Gaspard and Thaïs to their grandparents and left the nurses to mollycoddle Azylis. We've put aside our problems and ordeals and exhaustion, and run away from it all for a few hours. Carefree and happy. We followed the dramatic *route des crêtes* coast road before delighting in a stroll through the tiny streets of Cassis.

Now the day is coming to an end tucked away in the beautiful *Calanque de Sormiou* inlet. Protected by the rocky hillsides, it feels like the ends of the earth, with only the vast azure expanse of the Mediterranean as a horizon. What peace! I lean against a warm rock and make the most of the last rays of sunlight, letting the regular sound of the waves lull me. Loïc is half asleep beside me. I close my eyes. Slowly, the events of the last few weeks play out again in my head. And for once I don't stop the spooling images that are usually so painful. I let a new feeling spread through me: pride.

The poster for a charity operation called "To each their own Everest" makes its way into my thoughts. It hangs on the wall of the pediatric hematology unit. I walk past it every day. Every time, I sense my heart constricting a little, as if slightly discouraged. Yes, it's certainly true; we each have our mountain to climb. Only a few months ago, ours looked set to be an accessible, comfortable, privileged ascent—which made the fall all the more brutal.... Our path actually went off toward steep ravines, vertiginous cliffs, treacherous hidden dips, and unexpected pitfalls.

Today, after six months of this really trying climb, we're allowing ourselves a well-earned break; for a while, this rocky inlet serves as a mountain refuge. And I can finally turn around and look at how far we've come. What I see takes my breath away: We've covered all that ground already! I look back at it from a safe distance, following every twist and turn. The double blow of the girls' illness, the unbearable waiting, the sleepless nights and bleak days, Thaïs's pain, our leaving for Marseille, the girls being hospitalized, Azylis's transplant, the separations, Gaspard's tears, the emotional bruises. Our hearts broken so many times ... and yet we've survived. Despite the temptation, we haven't given up.

We've simply changed our strategy. We've stopped trying to make out the summit hidden in the mist; we've carried on little by little, cautiously, one foot in front of the other. One day after another. And we've come this far, closer together than ever.

I'm proud! Of us, of him, of our children, our faith and our love. Yes, I'm proud of our life and of all of them—everyone who makes up the long, silent, supportive rope that stays with us on this perilous climb, never wavering or giving up. They support us, some directly and others discreetly, they steady our footsteps and reinforce our achievements.

Now I know. I know with unshakeable certainty that one day we'll reach that summit way up there. All of us together. Way beyond the clouds.

S HE HASN'T LOOKED AT ME. MY HEART LURCHES. THAÏS IS lying ON her bed, silent and with eyes wide open. I move a little closer. Her eyes don't follow me. The evidence hits me like a physical blow: Thaïs can no longer see.

I'm floored by the violence of this shock. I stumble, try to catch my breath, grab hold of the sheet to stop myself going under. I'm disoriented, lost. Words fail me; not a single sound has the courage to come out of me. Thaïs blind, I can't believe it. . . . It's one of the stages I most dreaded. And it's happened already. I'll never get used to it. Never.

I run out of the room, I want to scream through this pain alone, away from her. I don't want her to see me in this state, even if she can no longer see. I collapse on my bed, inconsolable. I call on Heaven, begging it to give my princess back her sight. "Just her sight, please, just her sight." I stay there prostrate for a long time until I gather some of my strength. I have to go back and face those eyes that can no longer see.

I push open the door with the secret hope that I was wrong; perhaps she'll look at me as usual. If only . . . She turns toward me, but her eyes don't find me. I hug her to and speak into her ear.

"I'm here, my darling, it's mommy. Don't be frightened."

I rock her to calm her fears and ease her pain. But what fears? What pain? She doesn't look tortured. I now notice how peaceful she seems. It's my heart that's going to burst, not hers.

In my gloomiest nightmares, I imagined how distressed Thaïs would be when she was deprived of light. I pictured her in anguish because she was condemned to darkness. I went to great lengths to console her, but she was still desolate. Reality is taking a completely unexpected turn. Thaïs hasn't changed. Nothing about her suggests she's suffering because of this sudden blindness. She's the same little girl as the one who could see. If I hadn't tried to catch her eye, I might not have realized she was blind.

Over the last few months, I've read Thaïs's every emotion in her clear-eyed expression. In it I've often read amazement, pain, determination, pleasure, concentration, or happiness; but I've never detected an ounce of despair. She's always had faith and carried on along the path that's been carved out for her. A mysterious Princess Courage who'll never stop surprising us ...

I need to know, to be sure. When I looked deep into Thaïs's eyes, I always used to see a spark of life. I bring my face up to hers until I touch it, and slightly anxiously, I delve into her big black eyes. I can see it, the fierce bright little flame. It's dancing. "I'm here. I can't see, but I'm still here. Life goes on." She gives me new hope, filling me with energy and courage. That light is a shard of Thaïs's soul. A line from *The Little Prince* nudges into my thoughts, gentle as the wink of an eye: "We can only truly see with the heart. What really matters is invisible to the eye."

In a marathon, the last kilometers are said to be the hardest. Here too the last stretch puts us sorely to the test. Our tribulations in Marseille are coming to an end, but we're struggling to cover the remaining distance. I'm not even sure we'll all get over the finish line together....

I had secretly thought of the holidays around Halloween as the deadline for our exodus. I can see them striding toward us, and there's nothing to imply we're about to leave, because we have to come to terms with a complication: Azylis still won't take her bottle.... Since she moved to the protected area, we've tried progressive steps toward teaching her to suck again. Vain hope; she manages to swallow just a few drops in every meal.

The doctors have spelled out the problem clearly: So long as Azylis is dependent on a drip and isn't putting on weight, she can't leave the hospital. They're not actually worried, though, and have assured us it's a matter of weeks, a month at the very most. But we don't have that sort of time to play with. Not in Marseille, anyway.

Our plan, which has worked smoothly so far, is wavering and threatening to fall apart. Chantal has come home from her summer trip to the mountains. She's still just as welcoming and has invited us to stay as long as we need, but we don't want to inconvenience her in her own home. We've abused her generous hospitality long enough.

Loïc will have to return to work; he's expected in Paris in the next few days and can't stay on in Marseille forever. Both our sets of parents soon have to take up other commitments elsewhere. The scaffolding that was maintaining our fragile equilibrium is breaking up.

I've turned the situation over and over inside my head before facing the facts. We don't have endless different options: We'll have to be separated. The easiest thing would be for Loïc to go back to Paris with Thérèse, Gaspard, and Thaïs, while I stay in Marseille with Azylis for as long as it takes. I could move into a room in the Parents' House right next to the hospital. The two of us would join the rest of the family when everything has sorted itself out. This arrangement isn't very complicated to set in motion logistically, but it's unimaginable in emotional terms.

We need to be together to be strong. "One for all and all for one": We've adopted the Musketeers' motto as our own, even more so in the last few weeks because Thaïs is still going downhill; the regressions are often tiny, almost imperceptible, and sometimes devastating. Not one of us can agree to being parted from her at the moment, even if the separation is temporary. You never know what might happen.... . One month isn't much on the scale of a lifetime. But in Thaïs's case, it might represent an important proportion of her life. Her months are numbered. Time is short.

Another battle to fight.

ROLL ON PARIS! WE HEARD THE NEWS THIS MORNING: WE'RE all going home together! After much discussion, the doctors shelved their reservations about Azylis's leaving so soon. They let themselves be persuaded by the good results from her latest tests and a few mouthfuls of milk swallowed with a semblance of appetite. They've swiftly contacted a Paris hospital to ensure that the progress of her transplant continues to be monitored.

Our bags are packed and shut in the twinkling of an eye. The administrative formalities are dealt with. The final medical recommendations to help settle Azylis at home are taken on board. Our Marseille epic is coming to an end.

So here we are on our way home, feeling emotional about this turning point. We leave Marseille behind, along with so many dear people, family who are now closer than ever, nurses who have become friends, and "copaings." No more trips to school lined with southern pines and palm trees, sunshine warming our bodies and souls, late night suppers by candlelight in the dew, nights shoehorned into a hospital armchair, days in face masks and coveralls, Gaspard's expeditions in the garden, plus Ticola's arrival, Azylis's first gurgles, Thaïs's last looks; in short we're leaving behind a myriad of memories, bitter and sweet, times of tears and laughter. Not without shedding a tear.

Paris is opening its arms to us. We can't wait to get back to our apartment, our normal bearings, our little ways, our daily life ... the last packing boxes to empty, pictures and curtains to hang, and the huge amount of cleaning that's waiting after four months away!

Home, sweet home, here we are. All five of us. At last. There's a wonderful surprise waiting for us at the apartment: While we were covering the distance from Marseille to Paris, a battalion of good fairies infiltrated our home armed with brooms, brushes, floor mops, and sponges. They've polished, scrubbed, vacuumed, and tidied tirelessly for a whole day. The result is remarkable; there isn't a single sign of a whole season of dust.

A bottle of champagne is waiting in an ice bucket with one word written in bold letters on an improvised sign: *Welcome!* It feels so good to be home ... such a simple pleasure.

Gaspard can't contain his delight. He takes out all his toys, marveling at each rediscovery as if seeing them for the first time. Thaïs lies on her specially adapted bed, joining in with a smile. She found the journey very tiring but seems happy. Azylis doesn't see much of this wave of happiness washing over us. As soon as we arrived, we "cloistered" her in her room. It was one of the conditions on which she came home.

Her quarantine should last several months, giving her immune system time to develop and provide her with effective protection against the dangers of germs and viruses. For now, her only authorized outings are weekly trips to the hospital to monitor the transplant's progress, chart her blood cell production, and ensure she hasn't caught any infections.

Her room at home has been transformed into a protected area. It's been scrubbed from top to bottom and now has a strong smell of bleach and antibacterial gel. A smell we find reassuring. We're just as draconian as we were in the hospital: Before going into her room, we disinfect our hands, remove our shoes, and put on masks. It's not as restricting as at UPIX, but we have to keep up our vigilance because these sorts of practices aren't natural at home. We have to think through our every move. As an extra precaution, Gaspard and Thaïs aren't allowed in her room. This evening, though, we agree to slightly bending the rules in honor of this great day. We sit them in the doorway to their baby sister's room with masks over their noses. Thaïs is safely ensconced in her molded seat, and Gaspard is holding her hand, laughing nervously. Azylis sits in her cot, watching them with a hint of amazement. She doesn't recognize them; she doesn't actually know them. Not yet. For the first time in months, our three children are together in the same room. Or nearly.

The visit doesn't go on forever. Gaspard, Thaïs, and Azylis are very tired after a day filled with emotion. The moment they're in bed, sleep carries them off in its welcoming arms. Once the house is asleep, Loïc and I crack open the champagne and drink to our reunion as a family. Never guessing it will last no more than one evening. If we knew ...

It's a rude awakening. With the first light of dawn, Thaïs is vomiting, coughing, choking, and convulsing. Alerted by Gaspard's screams, we run to her bedside. I take her temperature, and the thermometer climbs above 104°. We don't waste a minute and drive her straight to the hospital department that monitors her. The doctors diagnose gastroenteritis complicated by a serious pulmonary infection. A veil has fallen over the future.

Our happiness as a family of five is over. Loïc is going back to work in two days' time, Gaspard is embarking on two weeks of school holidays, and Thaïs is in the hospital in critical condition. Our family nucleus has only just been reformed, and it's splintered once more.

I'd like to know one thing: Did Sisyphus rant and rage and drum the ground furiously when the rock he'd so laboriously rolled to the top of the slope crashed back to the ground? Or did he just return to his rock, unruffled, and resume his ascent as if nothing had happened? Indefatigably?

We don't have time to find an answer or feel sorry for ourselves because our peace has been so summarily interrupted. We pick up the pieces and try to restore a makeshift balance. Gaspard will spend the holidays with his cousins. Thérèse and I will swap duties between the two girls, one at the hospital, the other at home. Loïc will replace one of us in the evening when he comes home from work. It can work like that, we've already tested it out, not that long ago. We should manage this time too. At least for a few days.

M ONDAY, EARLY IN THE MORNING. AN AMBULANCE COMES to pick up Azylis to take her to the hospital. We're both ready, safely protected behind our masks. This first contact with the outside world makes me secretly nervous. Please don't let some malicious germ cheat its way into our trip. The ambulance crew are used to high-risk transfers; they're extremely vigilant. Azylis has nothing to fear. She's not worried about any of this anyway. She's enjoying the outing. During the few minutes of the journey, she tries to catch glimpses of the world that's denied to her. She cranes her neck to look out the window wide-eyed. When we arrive at the hospital, she's taken straight to a steril- ized room. She looks a little frustrated when the nurse closes the door, cutting her off yet again from the bustling colorful world outside.

We get to know the place and meet the medical team who will monitor the transplant's progress. The consultant checks over Azylis and outlines the schedule for her visits, treatments, and assessments. The next few months are going to be very busy: Azylis has to come here every week, and these appointments will be opportunities to ensure that everything is going well. On top of that, every three weeks she'll be put on a drip of concentrated antibodies to compensate for the deficiencies in her immune system. For all her other treatments, arrangements are made for her to have in-home care. A nurse will come over twice a week, mainly to change the dressing on the catheter.

The doctor points out that if she has the least sign of a fever, Azylis must be hospitalized. It's not thrilling news. A five-month-old baby has endless opportunities, often harmless, to have a slight fever. And if we have to bring her to the hospital every time she cuts a tooth, I reckon she'll be spending most of her time here. Still, we don't take this instruction lightly; one fever can mask another, perhaps from a far more serious source, such as a systemic infection carried by the catheter.

After a day spent in the hospital, Azylis is happy to be back in the ambulance, a source of unexpected pleasures. I can breathe a little more easily: I'm pleased with this first contact. To be honest, I was slightly dreading it. We were used to the staff and routines at the hospital in Marseille; here we have to go back to square one. It's not easy putting our faith in a new institution, however highly reputed it may be, and entrusting it with what we hold most dear. We'll see....

We arrive home at the same time as Loïc. I take a few minutes to fill him in on our hospital visit but don't go into much detail—I don't have the time. I grab a bag, throw in some overnight clothes, a good book, and a photo of the children and rush off to be with Thaïs. It's already dark outside, but the day is far from over.

A lioness's strength in a damselfly's slender body. That's what I see as I watch over Thaïs lying in bed: thin, ashen, and breathless but clinging to life and determined to fight. Since she arrived in the

hospital, she's had a succession of complications. The gastroenteritis is persisting, and the pulmonary infection is taking hold. She's
physically very weak but not giving up. She's fighting tooth and
claw to get through this difficult pass. It's going to take time, that's
for sure. Much more than for a normal child; her leukodystrophy
is darkening the picture. In spite of everything, I feel confident.
I'm sure she'll pull through yet again. Because she wants to.

This evening, though, her symptoms don't leave much room for
optimism. Her condition is deteriorating, her breathing slowing
down, her heart racing. The nurses stay in her room, doing more
and more checks of her temperature, cardiac rhythm, and oxygen
levels. They bring in more nebulizers and raise the oxygen output to
supplement Thaïs's chaotic breathing.

Shortly before midnight, when the doctor is about to request
a transfer to intensive care, the nurse picks up some encouraging
signs—the first for many long hours. Thaïs's pulse is slowing, her
breathing becoming slightly more regular. The storm is passing.
Thaïs didn't go under.

The next few days are critical, even with the barometer rising. My
little lioness very slowly gets some of her strength back, but she's still
very vulnerable. This bout has had an impact on her physical state,
an indelible effect.

Nothing will be the same as before. Thaïs has come home after
two weeks in the hospital. The infections are under control, but
Thaïs paid a high price. My Princess Courage expended a great deal
of energy overcoming them, with heavy consequences. Her condition has deteriorated further, and she's now subject to considerable spasticity (exaggerated contractions of muscles when they're
stretched). She can no longer cope with her molded chair, and she
grimaces with pain when we carry her in our arms or move her,
however carefully. The sentence is irreversible: She'll never get out
of bed again.

It's strange having two daughters, each in her own bedroom, separated from each other by a corridor they cannot cross. It's even more disorienting seeing their futures heading in such diametrically opposite directions. In a few weeks, Azylis will finally be able to cross the threshold and discover the world which has so far been hidden behind her bedroom door. She is signing up to a positive dynamic.

Thaïs, on the other hand, is gradually withdrawing. Over the course of her life, she has moved through every room in this apartment, first on foot, then crawling, and finally sitting in a special chair. She won't anymore. She will see only the aspects of life we bring home to her from beyond these four walls, beyond the rectangle of her mattress. Her world is restricted to six feet six inches long by three feet wide. Shrunken so small, it breaks my heart.

It's widely recognized that immobility causes all sorts of torments for body and mind. In terms of morale, Thaïs shows no signs of affliction. She lies peacefully in her bed, listening to stories, enjoying visits, and tussling with her brother. Physically, being bedridden raises concerns. Human beings aren't designed to live lying down. Thaïs experiences all sorts of discomforts: Her pressure points become inflamed, her limbs stiff, her bronchi congested. The situation can go downhill very quickly without swift action. To remedy this, the doctor recommends a daily visit from a physical therapist to facilitate her breathing and maintain a semblance of mobility.

We scour the Yellow Pages for a practitioner prepared to tackle this sort of rare condition in the home. The task proves harder than we first anticipated. We're on the verge of despair when we eventually find a precious gem: Jérôme accepts our request straightaway. When he introduces himself to Thaïs, she instantly takes to him although she can't see him. It's instinctive. I can feel her anticipating his visits every day. She sighs with delight when he comes into her room and lets him manipulate her with complete trust. It's very touching for me as a mother because, despite the changes in many of her faculties, I can tell that my daughter's heart still knows how to swell with affection.

An infernal downward spiral. Only a week after Thaïs came home, when she finally has regained her bearings and some of her strength, there are new complications. She's in pain again. Terrible pain.

The episodes are increasingly frequent and violent. Of course, we have a whole armada of drugs to give her relief, but the pain resists them, and the attacks are getting longer. They can happen at any time, with no warning, and end in the same way as they have started. They can be over in a flash or can go on and on for an hour. However long they last, they have one thing in common: They're unbearable. These excesses of suffering leave Thaïs exhausted and propel any witnesses into a state of shock.

This afternoon everything is calm in Thaïs's bedroom. She and I are huddled next to each other on the bed, listening to a story, when one of these attacks erupts—the most painful I've ever seen, the most traumatizing. I'll never be able to describe the scene. There's nothing worse than watching, powerless, as your child suffers. Nothing.

Never again. I never want her to suffer again. It's unbearable. We need to use more drastic measures, move up a notch, put every wheel in motion to ensure this stops. Right now.

Once Thaïs is calmer, I call the hospital. I'm still in shock, my fingers shaking as I dial, and my eyesight blurred by tears. When I explain the situation to the doctor, he decides to have Thaïs hospitalized immediately.

I have time only to gather the minimum requirements for a hospital stay, not forgetting the indispensable lullaby CD, before the ambulance arrives outside our building. A few minutes later, it's sweeping up to the hospital door, all sirens screaming. The journey has triggered another attack. I heard the driver commenting quietly, "Oh, my God, it's not possible to be in that much pain," before pressing his foot a little harder on the gas.

Zero tolerance. Confronted with pain, hospitals apply clear and precise instructions: On no grounds, under no circumstances, is a patient allowed to suffer. Even less so if it's a child. The thinking has changed: I remember when I was a girl having to grit my teeth and hold back my tears while the doctor assured me, "It won't hurt. Come, you're a very brave little girl." Well, yes it *was* painful getting all those stitches without anesthetic! He could at least have admitted it. In the past, they got rid of pain by denying it. That logic is now outdated. Thank goodness! Nowadays, not only is pain recognized but efforts are made to evaluate its intensity and suppress it, even in the very young.

The moment she arrives at the hospital, Thaïs is taken into the care of a female doctor who specializes in pain management. This is a new discipline in the medical profession. And oh, what a useful one! After a quick but thorough examination, she assesses our daughter's degree of pain; it's off the official scale. We already knew it was beyond intolerable. You only had to see her. . . . The doctor prescribes the necessary remedy to give her instant relief. Only moments later, Thaïs relaxes at last and gives in to restorative sleep.

Quietly, so as not to wake my sleeping princess, the doctor explains the pain relief system she intends to put in place. With the new approach to pain, medicine doesn't just acknowledge and ease physical suffering, it also tries to anticipate it. Thaïs mustn't have these episodes. Up till now, we were caught out by the rapid developments in the illness and the pain that went with them. From now on, we must be one step ahead.

The doctor reviews the whole array of analgesics that might be useful to Thaïs, from paracetamol to morphine, to nitrous oxide gas, the so-called laughing gas that blots out pain. There's no doubt about how effective these treatments are, and yet the doctor wants us to think before giving our consent, because these drugs are not without side effects. They're going to produce a marked sleepiness in Thaïs. That's the other side of the coin: She won't be in pain anymore, but she won't be so "there." We accept without a moment's hesitation.

"NINE THIRTY TOMORROW EVENING. BLUE WARD ON THE third floor, first room on the right. You're taking over from Caro. She'll give you the instructions. Marie-Pascale will take over from you at eight o'clock the following morning. I'll get there a little later in the morning."

"Okay. Got that. If there's a problem, may I call?"

"Yes, any time, day or night. Good luck and goodnight."

Anyone would think we were in a spy film. Reality is even more compelling than fiction. This is Thaïs's army in operation, an army that was assembled as soon as she entered the hospital. In fact, news of her hospitalization traveled more quickly through our circle of friends and family than a burning powder trail. Dismayed by this new separation, those close to us, and even those not so close, have offered their help and their time. A network is set up at lightning speed, taking turns to sit with Thaïs day and night. The principle is clear: We need to ensure there's someone by her side the whole time, twenty-four hours a day, relaying each other as much as possible. Sometimes visits overlap, when the relief guard arrives a little early or the previous visitor stays on. The nurses are used to this constant ballet of new faces beside our princess. They call it "Thaïs's solidarity."

Solidarity ... is that really what's driving these friends, relations, cousins, some young, some not so young, to spend an hour, a day, a night in a confined hospital room with a two-year-old girl who can no longer see, no longer talk, and no longer move? I don't think this is just a rush of solidarity, no. I can tell there's more to it. I can tell from how motivated they are that it's stronger than sympathy, more intense than compassion, deeper than affection.

Through anecdotes, personal stories, and confidences, each of them explains in veiled terms what it is that brings them to be with Thaïs. And we accept all their reasons—which boil down to just one—as gifts ... straight to the heart.

"Is anyone there?" The nurse comes into Thaïs's room and is amazed to find her alone on her bed, eyes wide open, laughing softly and turning her head from side to side. The cupboard door suddenly opens, and Caroline peeps her head out.

"Shh, I'm playing hide and seek with Thaïs. Don't say you've seen me; it's not easy finding a good hiding place in this hospital room. She finds me straightaway under the bed."

Touched, the nurse puts a finger to her lips as a sign of consent and goes over to Thaïs to administer her treatment as if there was nothing unusual. Thaïs is thrilled.

That day, despite being thirty, Caroline managed to find a childish spirit that had been buried deep inside her for too long. She found it for Thaïs ... and thanks to her.

Louis-Étienne is sitting on the edge of Thaïs's bed, his eyes red and his nose swollen. He's crying because his heart's been broken for the first time. At twenty, we're convinced the wounds inflicted by love will last forever and could even prove fatal. He's inconsolable. He confides in Thaïs, describing the torments of his heart and the vicissitudes of his love life.

Thaïs turns toward him, catches his attention, and starts to laugh. She laughs more and more exuberantly, without stopping—so loudly that Louis-Étienne can't resist the onslaught and lets himself be swept up in it. He starts laughing too. The two of them laugh a great throaty laugh. All of a sudden, he can look on the bright side again.

He kisses Thaïs's hand tenderly and, as if making a confession, admits, "You're right, little Thaïs, it's not as serious as all that."

Perhaps this is the magic that brings these cohorts of goodwill to Thaïs's side. The magic called love.

Happiness is sometimes based on such little things, tiny, minute. Ours takes shape this morning in a microscopic molecule: arylsulfatase A, the enzyme Azylis was missing ... and which is now present in her organism. It's invisible to the naked eye, but the tests are incontrovertible: It's definitely there! It's a beam of sunshine in the middle of December.

When Azylis was born, her level of arylsulfatase A was close to zero. She now has a normal level ... like someone who doesn't have metachromatic leukodystrophy. That was the whole point of the bone marrow transplant. We're there.

Having this enzyme is an essential prerequisite to halting the progress of the illness. Without it, nothing can stop the myelin being destroyed. We've taken a big step forward and suddenly embarked on a new course, one where we're allowed to hope. What if all this soon seemed like a bad dream? What if she starts walking when she's older? What if she can live like everyone else? What if, what if, what if ... I have a myriad of promising "if"s inside my head.

It's too soon to give a cry of victory. Far too soon. Nothing has actually been won, because although production of this substance is vital to curing Azylis, it doesn't necessarily guarantee that the illness will be curbed. Medical science can't explain the unfathomable mysteries of the human body. Not yet.

There's only one thing we can be sure of today: The enzyme is there. But there are still countless unknowns to confront. Will the enzyme be effective? And if so, will it be effective before the illness causes irreparable damage? Will it be sufficiently effective to stop the destructive process once and for all? Only time will tell. Every three months, Azylis will be subjected to a battery of tests to monitor developments as closely as possible. These tests will indicate whether her neurological and motor faculties are stabilizing or unfortunately ...

Fine, but that's not what's happening today. I'm leaving those worries for later. For now, I'm fully savoring the good news. As far as the future is concerned, I have to try to hope for the best by focusing on the positives. Things are making encouraging progress: The transplant seems to be taking very well, and the enzyme is there. That's enough to give us plenty of hope. And it's a recognized fact: Hope is life-giving.

"PUT YOUR WORK BACK ON THE LOOM TWENTY TIMES," THE poet Nicolas Boileau said, meaning things can always be fine-tuned and improved. Right now we're going under, overwhelmed by the terrifying increases in Thaïs's pain. It's ever more violent, forcing the doctors to keep reviewing their ideas and altering the pain relief treatment every day.

Thaïs has now been in hospital two weeks. She was meant to stay only long enough to establish appropriate medication, but her time here is dragging on and on. The picture is getting grimmer by the minute. Pain is no longer our only cause for concern, nor the worst; far from it. The illness is attacking the last ramparts. It's making inroads into her central nervous system and threatening vital functions.

This morning the doctor asked both Loïc and me to come to see him, a request which can't mean good news. When we're summoned together, it's usually a bad sign. This is no exception: In a colorless voice, he tells us that Thaïs's life is drawing to an end.

Already.

Winter permeates the room. Our tears freeze, our blood turns to ice, our hearts frost over. How can this be possible? I can picture my pretty Thaïs back in February, serenely getting on with life with her unusual little walk. That was yesterday! Since then the illness has gathered speed, galloping even faster than we'd feared. And there was nothing anyone could do to slow it down. Three brief seasons later, this runaway horse has unseated us, leaving us reeling.

In the summer, we already started worrying about how long she had, but not in the same way. Thaïs was very unwell at the time, yes, but she wasn't lost. Medical science could help her get out of that tricky phase. Today, now that we've reached this stage of the illness, we no longer have control of anything. Her vital functions could fail at any moment. Thaïs is at the mercy of fatal cardiac or respiratory failure. We're overwhelmed by a horrible feeling of impotence. What can we do? If we knew ...

Thank you, Don Quixote. His dogged battle against harmless windmills is an incalculable help to me. In these dark hours, it sheds light on one distinct point: You have to be sure you never identify the wrong enemy. Now there's one thing, sadly, that's absolutely certain: Even with the best will in the world, we can't save Thaïs. This assertion isn't an admission of defeat, it's just that I'm coming to terms yet again with the fact that, deep down, for months now, it's not leukodystrophy that we've been fighting.

This illness is a windmill which could make us flail the air pointlessly. We don't have the energy to waste; we surrendered our weapons long ago. But that doesn't mean we're standing by redundantly. We're trying to tackle another challenge. "Adding life to the days when you can't add days to the life." That's our fight. Not any other.

Back in the spring, I made a commitment to Thaïs in both our names, Loïc's and mine, to do everything I could to make her happy. That promise has more meaning now than ever. We'll carry on serving it. To the very last. And we won't shy away from anything.

It's now mid-December; Christmas is on the way. If there's one family celebration that Loïc and I particularly like, then it's that silent night. Ours looks set to be somber this year. It's entirely up to us to make it better.... Even without any discussion, we know what we want. We tell the doctor together: Thaïs is going to come home, for good.

It's madness! Yes, it's madness. Well, good! We're prepared to go completely mad for Thaïs's sake. We don't have the heart to entrust her final days to other people, in an impersonal hospital setting. She belongs at home, surrounded by her family. We feel we have the strength and courage to keep her with us. Nothing can stop us. The urgency of the situation gives us the impetus we need to take the step.

This leap into the unknown goes hand in hand with a giddying feeling that's both comforting and disturbing. Comforting because we're sure we're doing the right thing. Disturbing because we have no idea what's in store. Thank goodness.

The doctor accepts our decision and supports us by making arrangements for Thaïs to be cared for at home. In a few quick phone calls, everything's ready. We can go. When we leave the hospital with Thaïs, the nurses struggle to conceal their emotion. They know they'll never see their Princess Courage again.

In-home care. What a revolutionary idea. It can be summarized like this: If you don't come to the hospital, the hospital will come to you. Without wasting any time or leaving anything behind. The very day Thaïs comes home, a nurse rings the doorbell with a delivery to make Santa Claus and his legendary sack quail. It has everything: drugs, equipment, machines, pouches of food.

The in-home-care team is on familiar territory when it sets up in our home; the nurses have already been coming regularly to take care of Azylis. And I have to admit that more than once I made the most of their visits to ask them about a new bedsore, a sudden rash, a galloping heart rate. They willingly dealt with my anxious questions, but the situation wasn't very easy for them so long as Thaïs wasn't officially under their "jurisdiction." She is now. From now on, they have free rein to take things in hand. And they won't spare any effort.

Indispensible and temporary. In-home care can be encapsulated in those three words. It isn't a substitute for long, complicated hospitalizations, but is usually intended for patients on the road to recovery, giving them an opportunity to cut short or avoid a spell in a hospital. It is planned for a specific time period. A week, a month, perhaps two. But not much more.

Thaïs's case doesn't fit this pattern. With her there's no possible hope of improvement. No going back. No recovery. We can only hope for a reprieve. The deterioration in her state of health implies she will need in-home care for only a short time. But no one can predict the future, and the nurses know that. Just as they know what lies ahead for us. And for them. This doesn't put them off, quite the opposite: They like this slightly different approach to their discipline, this system of administering treatments not to heal but to make life more livable. Their commitment is unfailing; the in-home care will last as long as Thaïs lives. The nurses reiterate this as soon as they see any doubt in our eyes: "We'll stay with you right to the end."

In-home care makes our lives easier because Thaïs's life is in professional hands. It's a relief to see a medical team coming aboard our vessel. We can gradually go back to being parents rather than stand-in nursing staff. We can slot back into our proper roles, and things are much better like that. The nurses help us with bathing Thaïs, her treatments, and her day-to-day care; they evaluate her condition, chart its developments, and avert her pain. They act as an interface with the doctors, coordinate other professionals involved, and restock supplies of medication and equipment.

Every day without fail, come rain, wind, or snow, one of them comes to visit Thaïs. I get used to these daily visits. Better than that, I value them, look forward to them. A bond is being established, a solid one. Not in the same way as at the hospital, where the setting can create a degree of distance. We're at home here. We welcome each of them into our family unit quite openly. There's nothing they don't know about our bad days, our moods, the things tormenting us, and our pleasures too. They share our lives unaffectedly, discreetly, and affectionately because, of course, they become attached. How could they possibly not? You can't fail to become involved when you care for a sick person in his or her own home. Not one of the nurses disguises the deep feelings she has for Thaïs. They even sometimes come in twos to tend to her. The princess requires it!

Gaspard is standing in the doorway, his face downcast. Thaïs is moving out today. She's leaving their shared bedroom to move into ours. Instead of us. It will be better for her, and for him: their room had started looking like a hospital with oxygen tanks, bottles of pain relief gas, tubes, monitors, and supplies. The area meant for playing ended up considerably reduced.

Gaspard's mouth twists sulkily.

"I don't care about having room to play. What I want is to keep my sister with me."

As I dismantle the frame of our bed, I go back over the reasons for this change. The official reasons: how difficult it is to care for Thaïs in a small room, the constant coming and going, the sheer quantities of medical equipment, having to respect his sister's need to sleep, etc. Gaspard is not convinced, and he suddenly bursts into tears, saying "I want to stay with Thaïs, I want to stay with Thaïs" over and over. Only then do I find the courage to tell him what I wanted to leave unsaid.

The psychologist and the in-home care team recommended that we separate them, but it wasn't for practical reasons. At this stage in her illness, Thaïs's life is hanging by a thread. She could go to sleep one evening and not wake up in the morning. Gaspard knows this without having to be told. He doesn't even realize it, but he's watching over her. He interrupts what he's doing during the day to check whether she's okay. He takes a long time to get to sleep in the evening because he's listening to the machines. If he wakes in the night to go to the bathroom, he can't help checking that his sister's still breathing.

One morning, between two slices of toast, he came out with: "Mommy, daddy, if I wake up one morning and Thaïs is dead, what should I do? Should I come get you or not?"

My coffee mug slipped from my hand and broke, spilling all over the table. That was when we realized we urgently needed to change the setup.

Gaspard must categorically not be the first person to see Thaïs dead. That's not his job. It's ours. We made the choice to keep Thaïs at home whatever the circumstances; we have to take responsibility for that decision and arrange our lives so that everything happens for the best for everyone.

I explain all this to Gaspard in a version adapted to suit his age.

"We don't want to keep you away from her; we want to protect you so that you can go on living your life like a little boy."

"Yes but, mommy, that *is* my life, being with Thaïs. Afterwards she'll be gone, and I won't ever be able to see her again. Afterwards maybe I'll be a grown-up, and it'll be too late."

Yet again, I'm thrown by my child's sound reasoning, and it puts me back on the right track.

"You're right, Gaspard," I conceded. "Playing with your sister is part of your life. It's also a wonderful thing. But you shouldn't be responsible for her. We're going to go ahead and move her into our room, but you can come and see her whenever you want, day or night. You can stay here as long as you like."

Not a day goes by when Gaspard doesn't visit Thaïs. He often comes and sits beside her on her bed after school and tells her about his day. He laughs, and she smiles when he describes games in the schoolyard, the bread-ball fights in the cafeteria, and the teacher's reprimands. We're asked politely to leave when he tells her his little secrets, the ones we're not allowed to hear.

"I can tell Thaïs everything. It's handy, she never passes on secrets. And I'm sure even if she *could* talk, she wouldn't tell."

Sometimes Gaspard rushes into the room, gives his sister a quick kiss, and races back out. He goes into his room and closes the door, back in his own world. A world populated by dinosaurs with wise names, pirates armed to the teeth, valiant knights, and robots with superpowers. A world without leukodystrophy or bone marrow transplants or medical equipment. An innocent world fit for a boy of nearly five.

My head's in the stars. The ones twinkling on the Christmas tree in the middle of the living room. Gaspard's arms are laden with multicolored garlands as he enthusiastically finishes decorating the tree. He's humming appropriate tunes that he's heard from the Little Singers of Paris. *Silent night, holy night.* The mismatched shoes laid out in a half circle around the foot of the tree are slumping under the weight of beribboned parcels. The table is scattered with golden star-shaped sequins and the places are set, all in red and white. Thirteen desserts arranged on large, well-spaced plates, are waiting quietly for our eager, greedy fingers. It's nightfall; we light the candles and dim the lights. Christmas is coming.

Loïc's parents and sisters are here, joining us to celebrate Christmas. We promised Gaspard no one would look sad on this magical evening. We each have a bubbling flute of champagne in our hands as we throng around the tree, stationed beside our shoes laden with presents. Thaïs's and Azylis's are there too. We've put them here symbolically. I look at the carefully decorated parcels and feel a slight constricting in my heart. But no tears, I promise.

When the time comes for us to explore these longed-for gifts, Gaspard asks tentatively: "My little sisters ... couldn't we? Just for this evening. To be together." He's asking for a truce on this special night. Loïc and I exchange a look, won over by his request. Surely anything's allowed on Christmas night?

Thaïs is sighing on her bed and Azylis babbling in her room. Well behaved, the pair of them. With no idea of what's in store for them. In the living room, Zabeth and Armelle are making preparations for them to join us. They push the coffee table to one side, move the sofa, and free up some electrical sockets. Once everything is set up, they watch a very strange procession, more ceremonious than the arrival of the three wise men. Loïc comes in carrying Thaïs, as beautiful as Snow White in Prince Charming's arms. Raphaëlle comes close behind with the feeding pump. Pierre comes next with one bottle of oxygen and another of pain relief gas. I bring up the rear with Azylis, pretty as a picture in her scarlet dress. Yes, I took the time to change her into a party dress in honor of this improvised outing. Once a coquette, always a coquette!

We've decided to take Azylis out of her room on impulse, but that doesn't mean we've forgotten our instructions. We all disinfect our hands and put on masks. Azylis is wearing one too; it's meant to cover her mouth and nose, but it overlays her whole face. We settle her in a chair completely covered with a transparent protective layer. Of course, she doesn't want any of these precautions and concentrates on pulling off her mask. Successfully. In a matter of minutes, she's taken it off, crumpled it into a ball, and thrown it some distance away. This victory isn't enough for her: She pushes as hard as she can against the protective layer of plastic acting as a screen between her and real life. Soon, my darling, soon you can actually touch this world.

Three, two, one, go! The signal is given. We can open our presents. Gaspard can't wait any longer, complaining when the ribbon's too tight and tearing at the wrapping paper. He marvels over each new find with increasing enthusiasm. He alone makes more noise than the whole rest of the family! Loïc shows Azylis her new toys from a safe distance; they haven't been disinfected yet.

Christmas shopping for Thaïs was a real brainteaser. What can you give to a little girl like her? Tricky. She's not interested in dolls or jewelry or tea sets. I wanted to find things appropriate for her. In the end, I chose a perfumed candle and a CD of fairy tales. I open them for her, describing what I'm unpacking, and bringing the candle up to her nose. Her nostrils quiver. She can smell.. . .

Gaspard comes and leans against me, his hands loaded with treasures and his eyes shining with pleasure. The magic of Christmas spreads through all of us. After dinner, the party goes on to an unreasonable hour. No one wants to break the spell. When we're alone together, Loïc and I sit in silence for a long time, snuggled in a corner of the sofa, wrapped up warm in the depths of night. The bright stars are still twinkling. Not on the tree but deep in my eyes. It's my best Christmas ever.

The letter's there, folded, sealed, and tucked into Thaïs's health record. With these few words on the envelope: For the attention of the Emergency Department. This missive, signed by the neuropediatrician, was written a few days ago at our request. And a good thing too! It gives us much needed help this evening. When the ambulance team come through the door shortly after midnight, my hand shakes as I give them the envelope without saying a word. The emergency doctor opens it and reads it in silence. Once he's read it, he slips it back in the book, saying, "I understand." He goes into Thaïs's bedroom.

Thaïs is in a bad way, a very bad way. Her temperature is over 104°, but her hands and feet are freezing. Her pulse is at more than two hundred beats a minute. She's unconscious. While the paramedics busy around her, I open the letter and look through it myself for the first time. In it the neuropediatrician gives a summary of metachromatic leukodystrophy (not all doctors are familiar with this rare pathology). He retraces the successive stages of Thaïs's deterioration and makes a note of her current condition. He points out that the treatment she's receiving is purely palliative. He says that we understand the inevitable nature of the illness and underlines, twice, the fact that we don't want Thaïs to be intubated or put on a respirator. Lastly, he says that we want to be informed regarding how imminent the end is. The letter ends with one final recommendation: "Please do everything possible to relieve pain, which comes in devastating paroxystic attacks."

"Paroxystic" is the only word I don't know. The rest is clear. The doctor has described the situation perfectly and expressed our choices faithfully. Difficult choices that Loïc and I discussed at length. We made them with our hearts and conscience. The decisions are now mapping out what happens next and limiting what we can do: We want to be with Thaïs and to have her as long as possible, but without doggedly keeping her alive; we'll do everything to avoid her suffering but without curtailing her life. In other words, we simply want to respect the natural order of her time.

The emergency doctor perfectly grasps our decision, and he respects it. So he explains the situation.

"Thaïs is in a very critical state. Things could change at any moment, one way or the other. We'll stay here with you if that's what you'd like."

We gratefully accept their presence; it calms us.

Despite how serious the circumstances are, no one loses composure. The ambulance team relieve us from administering treatments, and the nurses try to lower Thaïs's temperature and steady her heart rate. They give her drugs, check her vital signs, and watch how these evolve. Loïc and I stay close to Thaïs, touching her, talking to her, and encouraging her to fight. Reassuring her of our never-ending love.

After two hours, her pulse slows a little and her temperature drops. The emergency doctor waits for these improvements to be established, then we all agree that the team can go. They prepare to leave, making us promise to call them back if things go downhill again. I see them to the door and, just as I'm closing the door, the doctor turns and says: "Congratulations for your bravery. The bravery I saw in that room and the bravery expressed in the letter." Then he turns away, visibly emotional.

At dawn, Thaïs wakes as if nothing has happened.

DECEMBER 31. THE LAST FEW MINUTES OF THE YEAR ARE ticking away. The takeover is guaranteed to happen, hanging by the hands of the clock, ready to tip into the unknown, just like us. We pass the milestone with a handful of people, our invincible, indispensable nearest and dearest. Those who dare to wish us a happy new year. The few.

Other people wouldn't risk it for fear of making a blunder, of saying something that will hurt us. Some don't say anything, prey to embarrassed silence. Others take a chance, backing away, stammering, and floundering. Through their clamped jaws we can just make out the words they've weighed up and chewed over. Hard to digest. They hope "that things get better this year, if that's possible." Better is the enemy of good … and my enemy too.

If you knew … I wish I could beg you all, on my knees if need be, to wish us a good and happy year. You who've tirelessly given us your support; you who constantly regret how powerless you are to offer us relief. Here's something that really would be of help today: Help us to get a foothold in hope! Do something to make us keep faith! Urge us to be positive!

More than anything else, we need hope and optimism. They're vital. You can start right now by wishing us a happy new year. And, please, lose the affected voice, the formal tone, the pitying looks. Wish it for us with all your hearts. Not just once but a hundred times. When you're worried you're overdoing something, you're not doing it enough.

We don't know when or how things are going to happen, but we do know what the next few months have in store for us. Yes, we know that only too well. We're not shying away from what is to come, but we don't want to think about it now. The time will come soon enough. If we focus today on what lies ahead, we'll be paralyzed by it until it comes and annihilates us. Paralyzed by fear only to end up drowned in despair.

The worst is always a given. Okay. But the best can happen too, and it deserves consideration. So for this new year, please, don't wish us better or good, wish us the best!

There's nothing fairytale-like about our lives. Yet here we are surrounded by pretty princesses: one of them, Princess Courage who's turning into Sleeping Beauty; the other, the Princess and the pea, who regally rejects her feeds.

Azylis is enough to give the weighing scales the blues. She weighs no more than eleven pounds, which, at over seven months, puts her in the abyssal depths way beneath the average curve printed in health records. In fact, we've stopped checking her weight. It only disheartened us more and did absolutely nothing to influence her appetite.

She's drinking, there's no doubt about that. But toy-sized feeds that barely reach the one fluid ounce mark, if that … She struggles to finish them. We try every trick to get her to gain weight. As the quantity is inadequate, we go for quality: The dietician concocts cunning recipes to make her food richer, so that every mouthful has significant nutritional value. We also increase the number of feeds: Azylis has five feeds spread over a twelve-hour day. They're actually not that far apart because she drinks slowly, very slowly, appallingly slowly. Each bottle takes at least an hour. For one pathetic fluid ounce. So, from getting up to going to bed, we spend five hours shut up in Azylis's room, cursing away behind our masks for her to speed up the pace and take bigger mouthfuls, dreaming of seeing her develop a lusty appetite. Nothing makes any difference. Not our supplications, not distractions or promises or cuddles. We'll just have to be patient.

Ah, patience. A virtue with which we're inadequately endowed. Azylis's marathon feeds are pushing us to our limits. Loïc and I dread them a little more every day. I know perfectly well that Azylis isn't just being awkward and that her trouble swallowing is an enduring consequence of chemotherapy. Even so, I can't force myself to be patient. I have a horrible feeling I'm wasting time as I languidly count her tiny mouthfuls.

Thérèse comes to our aid, almost in spite of herself, because one of her key qualities is exactly that: patience. Thérèse has a radically different attitude to time.

She's amazed that we always seem to be chasing our tails, complaining when we have to be patient, and cursing long lines. Thérèse never feels she's wasting her time. Whatever she does, she gives it her full attention. And she feels that every moment of her life has a value. When she gives Azylis her bottle, she doesn't keep her eyes glued to her watch; she delights in this time spent with Azylis, not thinking about the level of the milk or the minutes ticking by.

The same goes for when she takes Azylis to the hospital. It's a well-known fact that in hospitals you often have to wait ... and for a long time. I'm soon muttering, getting irritable, and pacing up and down. Thérèse, on the other hand, sees this time spent in the hospital as an opportunity to meet interesting people, experience a new environment, and slow the frantic pace of her everyday life. For her, waiting isn't empty time; it's a state in its own right and can itself be a source of riches. Thérèse doesn't put her life on hold when she has to wait around, she carries on living, just at a different pace.

I watch admiringly as she does this, and persuaded by her view and by the serenity emanating from her, I decide to imitate her. A difficult apprenticeship, this patience business. It will take me several days, weeks even, before I reverse my tendencies and see the time spent on Azylis's feeds as special time spent with my daughter. I restrain myself to avoid thinking about all the things I could be doing instead. I try to live in the moment, calmly and gently. Taking my time.

This new approach, this precious gift from Thérèse, will be very useful to me in many aspects of life. Particularly with Thaïs.

As if our schedule isn't busy enough already, a stay in the hospital comes and introduces itself right at the beginning of January, between Azylis's weekly visits. This time not in the hospital that's monitoring the transplant but in the one that's dealing with the illness. It's an important appointment: The department run by the professor who specializes in leukodystrophies has asked to see her. The time has come to compare her state of health against the figures recorded immediately after her birth.

So Azylis is going to spend three whole days under extreme surveillance. It's a busy timetable: blood samples, MRIs, lumbar puncture, nerve conductivity tests, auditory evoked potential. In other words, a whole bunch of tests that don't mean much to me but should say a great deal.

I wasn't expecting her reaction. I knew from experience that Azylis didn't mind being in a hospital. She's already spent so much time there that it's become a part of her life, and she always accepts it quite naturally. But this time it's completely different: Azylis experiences these seventy-two hours of hospitalization like a holiday camp! She's radiantly happy at the sight of a new room, new toys that are inevitably more interesting than her own at home, and new nurses, who may well be hidden behind masks but are only too ready to make a fuss over her. All these novelties are opportunities for delight. The tests are intrusive and painful, yet Azylis doesn't throw a fit about them. She cries just long enough, no more, then starts smiling again and making the most of all these new things she's discovering. And seeing her blossoming like that, I too forget what's at stake while we're here.

We're both captivated trying to put together a wooden jigsaw puzzle when the doctor comes in, closes the door behind him, and announces the news: The illness has not developed over the course of the last six months. The results still show a slowing in the central nervous system, but no more than in July. As for the peripheral nervous system, it's intact. Against all expectations.

I can't find the words to express my happiness, just like there were no words to describe my pain. The doctor doesn't say anything either, happy just to smile as he savors the good news.

We are all well aware that these good results don't guarantee Azylis's recovery. They don't mean things won't change for the worse in the future, but for now they're the best we could have hoped for. For nearly a year I've been forcing myself to live from day to day. So right now I won't think about what could happen later; I'm just going to make the most of this wonderful moment. I go back to playing with my daughter.

I TAKE A DEEP BREATH, CLOSE MY EYES, CLENCH MY FISTS TO give me strength. And here I go:

"Gaspard, I have some bad news for you. Ticola's passed away."

"What does passed away mean?"

"It means he's ... um ... that he's left us, he's gone away."

"Has he run away? Where is he now? When will he come back?"

"He won't come back, Gaspard. He's ... um, well, he's ... dead."

"Ticola's dead? Dead forever? Oh no, mommy, that's so sad."

The new year's starting with tears: Gaspard crying over his faithful companion's death. He hasn't seen him for several months because Ticola didn't come back to Paris with us. Having him in the apartment was incompatible with the hygiene requirements for Azylis, so Ticola moved to Loïc's parents' house in Brittany. Gaspard grudgingly accepted this separation for his sister's sake and was hoping to see Ticola again soon, when the next school holidays came along. But the change of climate from the warmth of the Mediterranean to the wet Côtes d'Armor proved fatal for the little guinea pig.

Gaspard's tears dry up along with his grief. He wipes his eyes with the back of his sleeve and looks at me, frowning.

"Mommy, why didn't you tell me straight away that Ticola was dead?"

"But I did tell you, Gaspard, as soon as I found out."

"No, I mean why did you say he'd gone away? It's weird. You knew he hadn't gone away because he won't be coming back. But you still said it."

"Yes, that's true, but I was worried about telling you he was dead. It's a difficult word to say, at least it is for grown-ups."

"We'll I'd rather be told 'he's dead.' *I'm* not scared of death. Everyone's going to die. Death's not a big deal. It's sad, but it's not a big deal."

Why is it that we, the responsible, reasonable, wise adults, have lost this wonderful simplicity? We get tongue-tied with euphemisms, things left unsaid, and taboos. Out of a sense of propriety, or just fear, we banish words like "death" from our vocabulary. The word becomes unspeakable and unbearable to hear. And yet it's an incontrovertible truth. And Gaspard, with his natural spontaneity, reminded me of that. I wanted to spare my little boy by skirting around the words, but that distressed him. He didn't need me to protect him; he wanted me to console him. It's not the words themselves that hurt, it's the way they're said.

Our family will soon be confronted with a death oh so very much more painful and news so much more difficult to break. Thanks to this conversation, I now know how I'll tell Gaspard when the time comes. It will take a lot of courage on my part to use the real words, neither cagily nor too emphatically. But I certainly owe my son that. Now I know what I'll tell him the day Thaïs goes away ... sorry, the day Thaïs dies.

"You can kiss her." The sentence rings out with the same solemnity as on a wedding day. But this moment is more moving than a marriage. The doctor tells me this at the same time as giving me the results of the last blood analysis: Azylis now has an effective immune system. We can drop the masks. I wasn't expecting news like this when I came to the hospital this morning. It's taken me completely by surprise and overwhelmed me. Like a girl about to have her first kiss.

A bit shakily, I take off my mask. Azylis stares at me, puzzled, then her chin suddenly starts to wobble and her eyes mist over. She stares at me intently. She doesn't recognize me: She hasn't seen me without a mask for more than six months. Almost her whole life. Not me nor anyone else for that matter. She doesn't know what a mouth is, or a nose. All she knows are eyes.

I catch her eye to reassure her, talking to her gently. The doctor reiterates his invitation.

"Go on, kiss her."

"Here, now, straightaway? I'm not ready."

"Of course you are, come on, you can do it. She's a bit confused, it'll comfort her."

It may seem ridiculous, but I feel shy. I've dreamed of this so often over the last six months. I take her in my arms, and when my lips touch her soft cheeks, my heart is unleashed. I'm like a bulimic giving in to a binge: I can't stop myself now, I consume her with kisses.

Azylis calms under this avalanche of kisses. With gentle little movements, she strokes my cheeks and mouth as if they were fragile, otherworldly. Then, laughing, she grabs my nose, my lips, my chin, kneading and pulling and twisting. She's no longer frightened, as if suddenly remembering all the kisses we gave her when she was a newborn. There's nothing better than a kiss to tell someone you love him or her. And to know you're loved.

I come out of the hospital to call Loïc and let him know about this event. The moment he picks up, I yell into the phone, "I've kissed her, I've kissed her!" Passersby stare at me, partly amused, partly taken aback. If they knew ... Oh no, I won't be forgetting that kiss anytime soon.

It's the butterfly effect. How one small event can trigger major consequences. Azylis's now normal immunity will have repercussions throughout our family life. It dawns on me as we head back home: The quarantine is over, Azylis can leave her bedroom, she's free to come and go as she pleases in the apartment.

She has so much to discover. And not a minute to lose. I open the door, drop my bag and coat on the floor in the hallway, and take my daughter on a guided tour of the premises. She's fascinated by this world that's finally being revealed to her, scrutinizing every texture, every color, every item. She doesn't know where to look; she wants to see everything, grasp everything, touch everything, as if catching up on the months of isolation and frustration behind her always closed door. Or as if she wants to store up a maximum of sensations before finding she's shut away in her room again. She doesn't yet know that that time has passed, that she now has her whole life to enjoy this. Her whole life.

The new discoveries don't end there, not by a long way. I've kept the best for last. I slow down as I reach Thaïs's room. Excited by so many new experiences, Azylis is squirming in my arms. I pause in the doorway, take a deep breath, and go in.

Azylis stops wriggling, stares at her sister lying in bed, and flicks a look of surprise at Thérèse sitting beside her. I come right over to Thaïs; her heart rate suddenly accelerates, and she opens her eyes wide; she can feel that her little sister is there. With a slow, infinitely gentle gesture, she half opens her hand. Azylis leans forward, frowning and serious. She seems to be delving through her mind, trying to find a particular memory. All of a sudden, she takes her big sister's hand and doesn't let go. Thaïs and Azylis recognize each other.

I leave them like that, hand in hand, their faces turned toward each other, in Thérèse's safe care. Gaspard needs picking up from school and doesn't yet know the good news. On the way home, I tell him there's a wonderful surprise waiting for him at home.

"A new guinea pig?"

"No, even better."

"I can't think of anything better. If it's not a guinea pig, I don't think it can be that great."

When he sees Azylis settled in Thérèse's arms next to Thaïs, he wails: "Be careful, you forgot your masks! And Azylis isn't even in her room! What's going on? This is all wrong. What a disaster!"

But there's no disaster here. Quite the opposite. I explain that everything's fine and Azylis no longer needs to be kept apart from everything.

"Are you sure?" he asks, perplexed. "Absolutely sure?"

"Absolutely sure," I tell him.

Then Gaspard gives a triumphant yell, lunges at Azylis, and hugs her in his arms, crying with happiness. I realize just how much he's missed her ...

Loïc finds us all like that, cooing around Azylis. He smothers his daughter in kisses, all the kisses that have been suppressed for months. What a lot of intrusions into her personal space that's been so carefully preserved until now! But Azylis isn't complaining, she's savoring every kiss. And she laughs with delight when her velvety cheek rubs against the rasp of her father's.

From then on, daily life becomes much more straightforward, for everyone. We all have a sense of newfound freedom, and we make the most of it, often gathering in Thaïs's room, just for the pleasure of being together.

Gaspard, Thaïs, and Azylis get to know each other. Over the course of these visits, the two sisters develop a wonderful complicity. Gaspard is very taken with Azylis, spending most of his time with her, and always reminding her she mustn't get upset if he leaves her because he'll be right back.

Azylis makes rapid progress now that she has contact with other people. She even starts taking more interest in her bottles as she sees us eating too. Loïc and I are glad to turn this corner, even though our reflexes have a hard time getting adjusted. There's no telling how many times we go over to Azylis without a mask and have a horrible feeling we've forgotten something important.

There's a spring-like warmth hovering in the air. A tentative sun seeps through fluffy clouds, and it's enough for us to forget the winter. This impression of spring gives me the courage to step outside with Azylis in her stroller, without any protection. Today is her first official outing.

She opens her eyes wide in amazement, contorts herself to watch passing cars, follows passersby with her gaze. She avidly devours all these new experiences and tilts her head toward the sun's warm rays. A light breeze takes her breath away. She inhales deeply, trying to catch her breath, and her little nostrils quiver. She's just met the wind.

Walking behind her, proud as Artaban, I steer the stroller, my face flushed with pleasure. This walk in the fresh air invigorates me, mind and body. I had to wait eight months to have this small pleasure again. Eight long months, almost a whole pregnancy. As if a new life were beginning today for Azylis, and for us. An ordinary life, the one we were hoping for.

People on the street hurry along, heads tucked between their shoulders, eyes pinned on the sidewalk. I'm surprised by this speed; I don't have the same urgency. I take slow, steady steps, savoring every moment of this outing. These are magic, floating moments, inflated with elation.

I walk along the middle of the sidewalk like a conqueror. A few passersby grumble, cursing as they step aside, bump into me, or overtake me. It doesn't get to me; their recriminations ricochet off my bubble of happiness. I'm taking my little girl out for a walk, and that's the only thing that matters. The world can stop revolving, it's all the same to me. Once around the block is enough of a pleasure for me. I feel like any other mother pushing her stroller, but with one important difference: I'm conscious of the incredible good fortune this constitutes, the simple act of taking your child out, quite normally, head held high.

*C*APILUVE. IT'S A STRANGE WORD, AND AN UNUSUAL PRACTICE. It's straight out of medical jargon and describes the technique for hair-washing when someone is bedridden. Since Thaïs has had to keep to her bed, we've learned the art of *capiluve*. Several times a week, with the nurses' help, we undertake this painstaking ritual ... to Thaïs's absolute delight, because if there's one form of care she likes better than any other, it's definitely this. It's such a delicate, gentle process.

Thaïs starts smiling when she hears us preparing the basins, bringing in pitchers of warm water, and laying out towels, brushes, the hair dryer, and hair slides. She quivers with impatience as we position her across the bed, her head held firmly between the nurse's hands. She sighs with pleasure when the water flows over her hair, and purrs beatifically when agile fingers make the shampoo lather with their regular massaging. She delights in the feeling of the brush gliding over her hair and the dryer wafting her pretty curls. She ends up falling asleep peacefully, relaxed and elegant in her braids or bunches.

I love Thaïs's ability to capture every happy moment. She has an innate capacity for detecting and extracting nuggets of pleasure right at the heart of her pain. This means that most of her treatments are sources of happiness because all she remembers of them are the benefits. Like when we massage her to avoid bedsores. Thérèse is an expert at this; she can spend hours anointing that paralyzed little body.

Each of us makes a special effort with all of her treatments. They're becoming increasingly numerous and frequent, so there's hardly a break between administering her medication, changing her, washing her, massaging her, and boosting her oxygenation. We turn these necessities into pleasures: a hand on her cheek during an oxygenation session, stroking her arm while her blood pressure is checked, a stream of sweet nothings while changing her. Thaïs can sense all the love and tenderness in these gestures. Precious little pockets of happiness nestling where we least expect them.

Hearing. It was all she had left, a frail link maintaining a semblance of normal communication. It's over. . . . When the tray laden with utensils and drugs clattered to the floor, Thaïs wasn't startled. She didn't even blink, but Gaspard and Thérèse ran to see what the racket was. She can't hear anymore.

Yet again, I discover this deterioration almost by accident. Until then, she'd given no sign that would have allowed me to guess any sooner. As with every other time, it comes as a blow to me. But perhaps not such a brutal one as its predecessors, because I now have such confidence in Thaïs and her incredible ability to adapt. I've seen it before, when darkness invaded her sight without casting shadows on her heart. Today's silence doesn't surprise her any more than that darkness did. She's not frightened of being cut off from the world; she isn't now, and she never will be. She's already on to the next stage, abandoning standard means of communication and appropriating other more subtle methods.

Our five senses are a luxury, and we're all too unaware of the fact. We have to lose the use of our senses in order to appreciate their true value and to realize their limits. In fact, mastering hearing, sight, a sense of smell, taste, and touch is at once a form of riches and of poverty. Riches because the senses complement each other perfectly, allowing us properly to perceive the world around us. Poverty because when we have the benefit of all our senses, we make do with them alone. Every exchange is made through these natural, instinctive, and restrictive channels. We can't imagine it any other way. But surely that's all there is: We have ears to hear, eyes to see, a mouth to speak, a nose to smell, and skin to feel? I don't think so. That doesn't take full account of human nature and our visceral need to communicate, share, and understand.

As a child, I read Helen Keller's moving story; I really admired the degree of understanding and communication achieved by this young girl who was deaf, blind, and mute. Deaf, blind, and mute, a state now familiar to Thaïs. Except that, to complicate the situation still further, my daughter is almost completely paralyzed. But still, in her case as in Helen Keller's, her will redoubles her abilities. Nothing stops her. When her senses no longer respond, Thaïs finds an unhoped for means of reestablishing connections: She makes the most of the slightest movement, the tiniest sound; she uses the density of her skin, the warmth of her body, the weight of her hands, the beat of an eyelid. She transforms all of these into signs of life, and proves with every moment that she really is here and understands everything that's going on. Thaïs is prepared to share what she's experiencing with us, but on one condition: We have to make the effort to meet her halfway, to receive her messages and decipher her codes. She needs us to listen out, not for her voice but for her whole being. And that's the secret: as an alternative to the luxury of the five senses, Thaïs offers us the riches of empathy. She's inviting us to develop our ability to sense other people's feelings.

I don't believe in spiritualism or telepathy. I believe in a dialogue between souls, from one heart to another, in communication through love. No, Thaïs can't see anymore, but she's looking; she can't hear anymore, but she's listening; she can't speak anymore, but she's talking. And she doesn't need her senses to do it.

E VERYTHING'S SO QUIET. TOO QUIET EVEN. I STICK MY EAR to the baby monitor. Not a sound … I jump out of bed, catching the bedside light at the very last minute as it topples perilously, and run to Thaïs's bedroom. I go over to her, feverish with concern, and crane to hear her breathing. I rest my hand on her chest. Her heart's beating peacefully. Her breathing is regular. She's just sleeping. Phew!

I stay a few minutes longer, watching her, then go back to bed. Loïc chunters, annoyed at being woken yet again. I look at the phosphorescent display on the alarm clock: It's four thirty. This is the third time I've been up tonight to check that Thaïs is all right, and sadly it won't be the last.

This scene is played out every night. However hard I try to reason with myself, I can't calm my fears. Since Thaïs has been back at home, since her days have been numbered, I have only one terror: that she'll die all alone, without a sound. That she'll need me and I won't know it. That she'll ask for my help and I won't hear her. So I've restricted my activities in order to devote almost all my time to her. I balk at leaving the room and walking away from her. I want to be there when the time comes. Of course, if there's an abrupt change in her heart or respiration rate, the alarms on the machines would alert me, day or night. But I don't trust them. They could happen to malfunction just as Thaïs is dying. Which is why I've set up the baby monitor connecting me to her when I'm not in the room.

The transmitter sits right next to her, a few centimeters from her mouth; the receiver is never far from me, going with me into the kitchen, the bathroom, or the living room. I only leave it when Loïc or Thérèse are at her bedside. Before I go to bed, I set the volume on maximum so I can hear her breathing. It soothes me and lulls me but also prevents me from giving in to a really deep sleep: I sleep with one eye and one ear open, with my senses still on the alert. The least sound or the least silence is suspect and wakes me. My anxiety builds up with each passing day.

As part of the in-home care team, a pediatrician who specializes in pain relief regularly comes to see Thaïs to evaluate her condition and her needs. This morning she notices the rings under my eyes, how pale and jumpy I am, and guesses that I'm worrying about something. I tell her what's causing my broken nights and admit that I'm keeping up an uninterrupted vigil. I feel tremendous trust in this woman, for her professional abilities but also as a person. We talk a lot, often about medical issues, sometimes about more personal things. Today she grasps my distress at a glance.

So, standing there beside Thaïs's bed, she describes her experiences as a doctor tending to children with cancer. Her voice is gentle, full of tact, respect, and propriety. She tells me about a little girl coming toward the end of her life, whose mother watched over her night and day, and who decided to die in the brief interlude when her mother popped out to buy a sandwich. She carries on with other similar examples. I look away: I'm beginning to see the moral of the story. And I don't want to hear it.

"Let your daughter choose." No, I can't do that. No, I don't agree. It's obvious to me that Thaïs wants me by her side at the crucial moment. How could that possibly not be the case? She's too little to go through this alone. And yet, deep, deep down, I can tell I'm on the wrong tack. I'm putting myself in her position, transposing my own fears. Thaïs may not be afraid of dying; she accepts events in her life so openly. She's already proved this to us so many times: She wants us to go on living and not put our lives on hold because of her. My constant presence is inappropriate; I'm being overbearing.

What if she wanted to be left alone? She can't tell us that; and even if she could, she wouldn't dare. No child would dare tell his or her parents that—it's too harsh ... and yet it's true. I know this but can't accept it. I want to graft myself onto Thaïs because if she dies when I'm not with her, I'll regret it for the rest of my life. I'll feel guilty for slacking in my vigil at that particular moment. I consider it my duty as a mother to be there. And yet ... I can't ignore the soft little voice whispering to my heart, "Let her live her way."

Yes, the doctor's right, one hundred percent right. I can't control everything, master everything. My little girl wants to be able to choose. I give in; this isn't an abandonment or a lack of love. Quite the opposite, it's one of the most remarkable ways I can prove my love.

My decision is made, although it pains me. I'm going to loosen my grip, a little, and try to go back to as normal a life as possible. It's the only way to move forward. Of course I'll still take care of Thaïs and watch over her, but not excessively. I hope I'll be able to. I'm shaking at the thought.

Good resolutions shouldn't be kept waiting; encouraged by the doctor, I unplug the baby monitor and stow it in the bottom of a drawer. Right at the bottom. Far, far away. That evening, I go to say goodnight to Thaïs calmly. I check her alarms several times and linger a while by her side, delaying the moment when I leave her alone. Eventually, I come out of her room but don't close the door. Once I'm in bed, I cock my ear and assess the silence. The only thing disturbing it is my stifled sobbing.

Everything's quiet. Too quiet? No, everything's normal. I can sleep in peace. More or less. Several times I have to battle with myself to stay in bed; I so desperately want to go and check that everything's okay. But I resist the urge. Day breaks at last. I stretch triumphantly. I did it!

We're walking on eggshells, or almost. When we go into Thaïs's bedroom this morning, we have to watch where we put our feet: The Easter Bunny snuck in here in the night. Easter is a major celebration in our family, rather more so this year than the last, in fact. Gaspard wanted to do the traditional egg-hunt outside, in the nearest park. We reminded him that Thaïs wouldn't be able to come with us if we went out, so he asked me if we could all be together in the living room like at Christmas time. We had to explain that it would be tricky for Thaïs, it would be better to arrange the festivities around her in her bedroom. He let us convince him out of concern for his sister, and because we promised him that, as a trade-off, he would get to hide some of the eggs, a privilege traditionally reserved for his father.

Gaspard certainly went to town: A pathway of little chocolate bunnies leads us all the way to Thaïs's bed. And there we find a display worthy of a demented henhouse. Thaïs is brooding myriad eggs, each more colorful than the last. They run all along her legs, trace the outline of her arms, nestle in the crook of her hand, and form a crown around her head. What a spectacular image! Thaïs is smiling, delighted by this invasion. Not far from her, an army of chocolate chickens is standing guard around her machines. One of them, the boldest, has come a little too close to the oxygen equipment and is starting to melt.

Gaspard is in heaven. He's realizing, to his delight, that he alone will be able to enjoy this haul. Which doesn't take into account Azylis, who, in a quiet corner, is tucking into a golden rabbit without going to the trouble of removing its foil wrapping. Is she getting greedy? Well, that *is* good news!

There's a happy atmosphere, each of us enjoying this moment of pleasure in his or her own way. At the end of this delightful day, I appreciate the cheerful Easter bells ringing just that little bit more. And I dread the knell that will soon sound in our house.

"No!" It's her first word. After "daddy," of course, but actually before "mommy." She could have said "sleep," "noonoo," "biscuit," or something else, like other babies. But Azylis definitely isn't like other babies.

As the days go by and she comes in contact with the world, she's revealing her personality. And what a personality! Azylis's character is an explosive mixture, a clever combination of determination and good nature. She knows what she wants. Always. And what she doesn't want. And when she doesn't want something, nothing can make her change her mind. She keeps on smiling but doesn't give in. Ever. Which is why no one's really surprised to hear that radical "no" coming from her. Not a shy no, a resounding one. Everyone's aware of how firm her decisions are; the in-home care nurses have nicknamed her "Miss No-No" because she often doubles up the interjection to make absolutely sure she's understood.

Driven by this will and her lust for life, Azylis is making her way in the world. Or rather gamboling through it. Seeing her getting on so well, there's nothing to betray the fact that she's faced so many trials since she was born. And yet her first ten months were more eventful than many entire lives. She seems to have come through all this without trauma. There's only one reminder that upsets her: masks. As soon as she sees someone in a mask, she's terrified. It seems to be her only bad memory. She shows no physical traces of the months in hospital. Her features, which were once bloated because of her medication, are back to their natural delicate proportions; her short sparse hair has grown again, the tips forming adorable, soft fair curls; her complexion has taken on a warm glow, hinting that she might be lucky and inherit her father's tanned tone; and the hard-won pounds have given her cheeks a delicious fullness.

Azylis has found her own place in life at home, taking part in all daily events. She doesn't miss a single visit, waiting for deliverymen and looking forward to the visits by the physical therapist and the nurses. As soon as anyone rings the doorbell, she crawls over as fast as she can. When the visitor's been identified, she goes ahead of him or her to Thaïs's bedroom. Once there, she reaches up her arms, asking to be put somewhere near her sister where she can see. Then she sits still, mounting the guard, to make sure everything is done in the usual order.

Azylis knows by heart what each person does with Thaïs. She watches closely, not missing a thing, and imitates them perfectly. She lifts the corner of the sheet to check that the sensor for Thaïs's oxygenation level is attached to her big toe. With a seemingly professional eye, she inspects the cover of the gastrostomy and how the feeding tube is attached. Then she checks if the oxygen tubes are in the correct position.

At times I feel Azylis is simply mimicking, without understanding or analyzing the implications of these details, like a little girl copying her mother by spooning imaginary food into a doll's mouth, or pretending to change its diaper. But there are times when she knows that what she's doing will soothe Thaïs: when she squeezes her hand to stop her shaking too much; when she wipes her mouth with a bib; when she presses her cheek against Thaïs's and buries her fingers in her hair. In these precious moments, Azylis is nothing but gentle. Then she reverts to her boundless energy and goes off to live her life. And she's happy, always happy.

I like routine. A year ago, I would never have guessed I would say that. Until now I've always dreaded being in a repetitive pattern. I sniffed out the least signs of one and fought them instantly for fear they might become entrenched. I made a point of creating a lack of rhythm in our lives. It's so often been said that routine is the sworn enemy of a relationship. I don't think that anymore. I now appreciate our humdrum daily life: It's proof that everything's going well. Let's make the most of it. It's a fragile balance, a precarious period of calm. For now, there's no major setback or life-threatening fear to shatter the peace. So we're savoring this drama-free, trouble-free blessing.

The key aspects of our schedule are well established. Thérèse is infallible, which is a good thing because over a period of six months she's become indispensable. The in-home care arrangements are perfectly set up. The nurses, four of them in particular, have every detail of what Thaïs needs at their fingertips. The oxygen tanks, feeding pouches, and other medical equipment are regularly restocked. The willing help offered by friends and family is still going strong, frequently giving us a break when someone watches over Thaïs for us. The physical therapist comes every day to help improve Thaïs's breathing; and, for some time now, Azylis has also been entitled to her own session at home twice a week, to help her catch up with regard to the slight delay in her motor skills accumulated during her months in isolation.

The results of Azylis's latest trimonthly checks continue to be encouraging. As her brother so rightly says, she's still getting good grades! There is a drop in her nerve conductivity, but it's so slight that there are no grounds for concern. Well, I hope ...

Gaspard carries on in his own sweet way, without a care. We can't get over how well balanced he is. He's happy at school, at home, at rugby, in life. He's never short of praise for his sisters who, in his eyes, are the prettiest girls in the world . . . and the only ones worthy of any interest, come to that.

Thaïs is staying on an even keel. Her days are all very much alike, sometimes disturbed by a spike in temperature, abnormal breathing, or an irregular heartbeat. But the crisis passes of its own accord every time, and life goes back to normal.

Loïc is fulfilled in his work; he's even forging ahead and nurturing new ambitions. That's a positive sign of newfound hope in the future. As for me, I'm gradually succeeding in establishing a balance at home, with a snippet of peace and hope.

Yes, routine's a good thing.

T HERE ARE SOME INTUITIONS THAT DON'T FAIL. A MOTHER'S
are infallible when her child is slipping away. I don't have to
wait for the nurse's diagnosis to grasp how extremely serious the
situation is. I don't need the frantic vital signs alarms to realize how
imminent the end is. On this sunny Pentecost Sunday, Thaïs is living her final moments.

The previous day, so easy and lighthearted, suddenly seems far
away. Yesterday, Thaïs woke with a cool complexion, breathing
peacefully. Everything looked so promising that we dared do something: We played truant for a few hours for a very special occasion.
Gaspard, Loïc, and I put on our smartest clothes and headed off
to celebrate Gaspard's godfather's wedding—without the girls. And
with no regrets or concerns; our daughters were in safe hands at
home with their grandparents who were pleased to have this time
alone with them.

The day went wonderfully well. We weren't very far from home,
ready to come back at the first warning, and of course we called for
updates two or three times, perhaps more. The answer on the other

end of the line was always the same, a reassuring "nothing to report, everything's fine, make the most of it."

Opportunities like that are few and far between, and all the more valued for that. So the three of us did the party justice late into the night. We slept in a hotel, prolonging our escapade into the following morning, long enough for Gaspard to taste every flavor of conserve at the gargantuan breakfast. We were home before noon, delighted by our celebratory break. And delighted to be reunited with our beloved girls.

The degree of emotion in our reunion implied it had been a long separation. We kissed Thaïs and Azylis as if we hadn't seen them for ages. Yes, sometimes twenty-four hours can be an eternity.... Azylis greeted us with a recital of spirited cries. Thaïs's enthusiasm wasn't as noisy as her sister's but still appreciable. We did the right thing going away, everything was fine in our absence. And we did the right thing not lingering too long before coming home, because shortly after we returned, the storm hit with no warning rumble or roar of thunder.

It's all over. Thaïs's heart is slowing with every beat. Her breathing is slipping into endless-seeming periods of apnea. We hang onto the silences between her breaths. Every inhalation could be the last. There's nothing more the nurse can say. She shakes her head to mean she's powerless, and tiptoes out, her heart in shreds, to respect the intimacy of this goodbye.

As the color drains from my adored daughter's face, all sense of calm is lost to me, all faith abandons me. I've prepared for this fateful moment, but I'm not ready. How could anyone be? My mind baulks and rebels and revolts.

No, not this. Anything but this.

Stay a bit longer, my princess, my Thaïs, my lovely! I can't let you go. I haven't the courage to go with you, and I haven't the strength to live without you. I'm clinging to your arm, your neck, your limp body to hold you back. Just a bit longer. A little bit.

Don't leave me. Not now. Not so soon. I want to keep you. Forever. To look after you, watch over you, cherish you, and love you. I never tire of you, your silences so full of meaning, your childlike smell, your soft, soft skin, your honey-colored hair, your half-open hands; all the little things, the sounds, the noises, the movements that are you. And that I love.

I beg of you, my little one. Hold on, fight. I'm nothing without you. You're my sunlight, my horizon, my gentleness, my strength, and my weakness. You're my rock and my rock bottom. My love.

Stay a bit longer, just for today. And tomorrow. And the next day.

Did she hear me? Was she aware of the desperate supplications from every heartbroken inch of me? I'll never know. Either way, Thaïs's soul has retraced its steps somewhere between heaven and earth and slipped back into the wearied body it was breaking away from.

Against all expectations, Thaïs is gradually coming back to life. One beat after another, one breath after another, she's climbing slowly, hesitantly back up the path, balancing on a fine tightrope. I don't slacken my grip or stop my supplications. Quite the opposite: As hope drives the ashy gray from her cheeks, I redouble my pleas.

It will be several trying hours before we conclude that Thaïs is out of danger. The nurse and doctor who arrive at this point heave a sigh of relief along with us. They know that the alarm was all too real. But the secrets of life and death are often beyond man and his extensive knowledge. No one, no doctor, however competent, no professional, however informed, no parent, however vigilant, no one can predict the day or the time. And perhaps it's better that way...

The ordeal of this imminent death, of this immeasurable suffering and the abyssal pain in the pit of my stomach could have destroyed me; but it will only make me stronger. And free me from a burden: No more good resolutions of heroism, stoicism, and bravura! I've stopped preparing for Thaïs's goodbye. It's a waste of time; I know that now. And that's not what counts: It doesn't matter how I react the day she leaves us. I'll be there as I truly am, just a mommy with all her suffering, all her fears, all her tears, all her weaknesses, but also all her love.

Loïc will be there too, I know that. He'll never be a deserter, despite the trials, like this afternoon's. When a heart is contorted with pain, a desolate loneliness sets in because it's impossible to imagine anyone else suffering as much—even the person crying alongside you. When Thaïs was dying, Loïc and I were aware of a divergence, each isolated in our own pain. He was the father unable to protect his child, I the mother unable to hold onto her daughter's life. A simple crack cleaved between us, a crack that could have become an impassable crevasse if we hadn't guarded against it. It takes more than huddling against each other to stay close. You have to find the strength, in the very heart of suffering, to dry the other's tears. To turn to that person and understand how he or she is experiencing the pain. We identified this disastrous fissure and repaired it—by loving each other, talking to each other, and listening to each other. By sharing each other's pain.

From here, more in love than ever, we need to take another step. Thinking we'd lost Thaïs forever sheds new light on our future. We saw her life deserting us; we're now going to savor every moment with her as a reprieve, a blessing, a priceless gift. I have to admit that, until now, as night fell every evening, I couldn't help but think, *We have one less day left with her*. Now, as it grows dark, I want to be able to say, "Today we had one more day with her." It's just a question of perspective, but it changes everything. We're going to make the most of Thaïs. Right up to the last moment. Then we'll have the whole rest of our lives to come to terms with her absence.

THE FLAME WAVERS, DIPS, HESITATES, THEN GOES OUT WITH a small plume of black smoke. Her face full of concentration, Azylis has just blown out her first candle, all on her own like a big girl. A pretty pink candle standing upright in the middle of a huge cake. Azylis is triumphant as we clap and cheer around her. Her smile glows with happiness and pride. Ours too. One year. She's already one year old.

You could summarize the first year of her life like this: a week of chemotherapy, a stem cell transplant, two blood groups, three months in a sterile bubble, four hospitalizations (per month), five different hospitals, six months in isolation, fifteen paltry little pounds, nine physical therapy sessions (per month), ten minutes to swallow each mouthful, eleven MRI scans, a succession of scans and lumbar punctures, twelve months of ordeal . . .

Or like this instead: one smile, two big mischievous eyes, three little teeth, four limbs crawling at top speed, fifteen good pounds, eight seconds standing without support, nine months at home with us, ten agile fingers, eleven hours of peaceful sleep (per night), twelve months of happiness.

Happy birthday, my beautiful Azylis!

The last days of June bring the school year to an end. Gaspard puts away his satchel and tidies away his books, pens, and pencils. He sighs with satisfaction, "Holidays at last!" I don't have the same feeling of relief. The advent of these two summer months has me perplexed: What are Gaspard and Azylis going to do with all this time? We also need a change of scenery, but we haven't made any plans so far. I should have taken care of it sooner, but I've kept putting it off for want of a satisfactory solution and the necessary courage. Thaïs's condition chains us to Paris. I could send Gaspard and Azylis to stay with their grandparents, but I don't really want to be separated from them. So how are we going to get out into the fresh air?

A plan is emerging, a slightly crazy one. Some very good friends have invited us to spend a week in Sardinia in July. The invitation's tempting but strikes me as far from achievable, particularly as Thérèse will be on vacation at the time. Who will watch over Thaïs? No, it's really not imaginable. Loïc doesn't see it like that and announces that nothing's impossible. He's not inherently wrong; it would be possible but difficult to set up. Firstly, from a practical point of view, we'd have to find volunteers to stay with Thaïs while we're away. We put out some feelers with friends and family, and our enquiries meet with unexpected success. Every person we mention it to gives a positive response, though not without imposing certain conditions: They want an exhaustive list of instructions for Thaïs's treatments, routines, and requirements. Loïc offers to take responsibility for the training program. With all his characteristic professionalism, he draws up precise instructions, written like a user's manual, complete with tables and a daily "route map."

With the practical aspects arranged, there is still one outstanding detail, and it's not a minor one: convincing each other. Of course we're sure of the benefits this trip will have, but it's so painful leaving Thaïs . . . the pain is psychological and physical. Like an amputation.

What were we thinking, what were we thinking going away like this, such a long way away? Without her! How thoughtless!

Gaspard is at the far end of the departures lounge with his nose pressed against the huge window, jigging with excitement: "Mommy, look at that plane there. It's huge! Look, mommy, look!" I don't get up from my molded plastic chair. I'm bogged down in misery, my stomach in knots. It's torture for me being away from Thaïs, knowing she's back there, in her room, sleeping on her bed, so beautiful, and not being with her. It's my duty to be by her side, not basking in the Italian sun. I have no right to go off like this and abandon her. What if she dies while we're away? Oh my God, what were we thinking?

Maybe it's not too late to cancel, turn around, and go home to her, quickly. I glance over at the window where Gaspard and Azylis are watching the choreography of planes. They look so happy.... .

Loïc turns toward me and gives me a wave. Seeing my ravaged expression, he comes over. He knows what I'm going through; he's feeling it too. "Be brave. We've made the right decision. We can't all stay in the apartment all summer, going around in circles. We need to make family plans and see them through. I'm sure that's what Thaïs wants for us. And for her. She wants us to stay properly alive. So let's make the most of this vacation. Let's live it to the full, with no regrets or remorse."

Someone once said life was a succession of separations—from birth right through to death. Some of the separations are physical, others psychological. Some temporary, others definitive. Some insignificant, others radical. Some gentle, others violent. Some a distancing, others an emancipation. Some a tearing away, some a tearing apart.

Learning to cope with life invariably involves mastering our autonomy. Who finds it more difficult to accept, children or their parents? It's agony being away from Thaïs, even for a short time. I've succeeded in releasing my hold a little by switching off the baby monitor one night and then the next. It's still painful. So flying across part of the Mediterranean without my princess is beyond my abilities as a mother.

How wonderful, I mean how wonderful to have come here! Sardinia soon dries my tears. You don't cry in paradise. This bewitching place is a complete change of scenery. The house is stunning, cool and white, nestled amid flowering vegetation, with views over a sea so blue it rivals the immaculate sky. Everything here is an invitation to a *dolce vita*.

The atmosphere is warm and relaxed. Gaspard has been reunited with his great friend Max, and they don't lose sight of each other for a moment. Azylis is reveling in the joys of a social life, playing the role of the princess before a court of children at her beck and call. She's never short of volunteers to pick her up, play with her, and feed her. In a word, she's in heaven. And we can really, truly catch our breath. These friends are worth their weight in gold, she is, he is, and their exuberant tribe. They spoil us and pamper us, surrounding us with treats and kindness.

This vacation is a blessing. I have to admit our batteries were nearly on empty. We wouldn't have held out long without this salutary interlude. We were starting to run out of energy, torpedoed by the lack of sleep and the constant tension. Here, freed of the constraints of daily logistics, we're recharging our batteries. And we're really sleeping, deep restorative sleep. With no jolting awake, no untimely disturbances, and no nightly fears. We arrived exhausted and stressed, about to touch bottom. At the end of this Italian week, we head home relaxed, rested, lighthearted, and tanned.

The news from Paris is good. The relay is holding out and the sentries taking over from each other without a hitch. Thaïs is doing well; she's being mollycoddled, spoiled, and fussed over by her guardian angels. Parents, sisters, cousins, they've taken it in turns to spend two days with Thaïs, two days to enjoy her. They clearly wouldn't exchange this time for anything in the world, and Thaïs herself is appreciative and doing well. In fact, it's amazing: There wasn't a hint of concern in the whole seven days we were away, which never happens in normal circumstances.

Yes, it really was a good idea to dare to go away, an idea that leads to others: We're now planning a possible week in Brittany toward the end of August. It's a good sign if we're starting to make plans, even small ones. We're freeing ourselves from our vision of life lived from one day to the next, and venturing a little further into the future. It does us so much good.

And so does coming home to Thaïs.

Plenty has happened while we've been away ... the nurses and our parents have hatched a real revolution.

We quickly get wind of the fact that something's going on. The day after we come home, the nurse starts asking us about our trip to Sardinia, about the benefits of having a change of scenery, and whether we'd like to do it again. My mom's smile speaks volumes.

They have it all planned. The only thing missing is our agreement. If we like, the in-home care team have arranged with my parents for us to spend the whole of August in my parents' house to the south of Châteauroux. And when I say us, I mean all five of us. This time Thaïs will be coming too. What a wonderful surprise! Unhoped for. Never in our wildest dreams would we have pictured going away with Thaïs. Sometimes reality outstrips dreams.... . Thank goodness!

"Don't you worry about anything," the nurse reassures us. "Everything's ready. All the arrangements have been made: The equipment rental company has already been told, the family doctor has agreed to take responsibility for monitoring her care, and there's a palliative care team ready to take over from us."

Our departure is scheduled for August 1. All we have to do is pack our bags and count the days. But a grain of sand slips into the cogs of this plan, threatening to compromise the whole thing. The Medicaid system has refused to cover Thaïs's transport by ambulance from our apartment to my parents' house; they see this as a nonessential trip. Their understanding of the situation is open to discussion, but this isn't the place. So what can we do? We have to move Thaïs by ambulance; no other means of transport would be conceivable. When the ambulance company tells us how much the trip would cost, we start despairing: The number has four figures in a row with no decimal point. There's nothing surprising about that; it covers the mileage cost, fees for a driver and a nurse, the medical equipment, etc. Our family budget can't take on this sort of expense. Yet can we let a financing problem threaten our wonderful plan? We have to find a way to put together the money. A solution comes to save us at the last minute, a solution hiding behind three generous letters: EAL.

EAL, the European Association against Leukodystrophies, a source of comfort and solace in our lives. The EAL offers support to families like us affected by myelin-related illnesses. Put another way, the association specializes in high-altitude expeditions: It helps us climb our daily Everests.

We first contacted them very soon after Thaïs's illness was diagnosed. It was a tentative first contact; we simply wanted to establish a connection and make ourselves known to them but didn't dare open the door wide. It was a difficult step for us to take; we didn't want to come face to face with other affected people, other suffering parents. We were afraid of what they might reveal and that the appalling reality of the illness would smack us full in the face. We thought we should spare ourselves that but quickly realized we should share experiences. Who better than other parents in the same position to understand our ordeal?

Amongst ourselves, the families in the EAL, there's a combination of propriety, respect, shared experience, and sincerity. Amongst ourselves we have no room for euphemism, we use the real words with no fear of shocking each other or being misunderstood. Amongst ourselves we're free to laugh, make jokes, and cry. Amongst ourselves there's never an awkward look or an inappropriate question. Amongst ourselves compassion assumes its full meaning and solidarity its full force. Amongst ourselves we make up one big family. A battered, amputated family, but a close-knit, united one. A wonderful family.

The EAL doesn't stop at forging links between families; in addition to moral support, it offers practical help. Finding that someone has an illness like leukodystrophy generates a multitude of often complicated and always tedious administrative processes. The EAL is on hand for this sort of thing too; its employees and volunteers are familiar with the administrative labyrinth; they anticipate requests, fill in forms, and steer applications. The association is also aware of the financial difficulties families may face, and it doesn't settle for easing their daily life but aims to improve it—by helping a family go away for a vacation with their little girl, for example. Their last vacation together.

Ten past eight. They're on time, a little early even. A good thing too because we've worn down our reserves waiting. We've been ready since dawn, excited and stressed by the day's big event: Today we're all going on vacation.

We open the door to two familiar faces: This ambulance team has already taken Thaïs and Azylis to the hospital several times. I recognize the driver who took Thaïs in an emergency when she was in terrible pain. And that's reassuring. I'm convinced they'll take the greatest care of my pretty princess.

It's a tricky moment: We need to transfer Thaïs into the ambulance, but she can't bear being moved; every movement is torture. The ambulance men have anticipated this problem and brought a mold which can be emptied of air to adopt the exact outline of Thaïs's body and hold her firm. Loïc watches the maneuver anxiously, compulsively repeating the words, "Gently, be careful with her, gently." Thaïs flinches and grimaces, only relaxing once she's secured in the mold. Every move the ambulance men make is controlled, and they walk very slowly out to the vehicle. Equally carefully, they lay Thaïs down onto a specially adapted stretcher. It looks like the hardest part is over. We can go.

I climb into the front, next to the driver, while his colleague takes up his position beside Thaïs, connects up the machines, and monitors her vital signs. Loïc leads the way with Gaspard and Azylis in a car filled to the gunwales. I can't wait for this journey to end and for today to be over. In the back, Thaïs is moaning a muted complaint. Her eyes are wide open, swiveling in every direction. She's distressed to be leaving her room and the world she knows. Attentive as a chivalrous knight, the ambulance man holds her hand, gently strokes her hair, and hums her a lullaby. Thaïs eventually falls asleep.

The miles go by, and the journey carries on calmly; we're getting close to our destination, and I let myself snooze. When the ambulance slams to a halt with a screech of brakes, the driver curses. Two cars ahead of us, a vehicle has left the road, somersaulting several times and crashing to a standstill on the shoulder. Our driver parks up immediately, and his colleague leaps out of the ambulance. In a few quick strides, he's at the scene of the accident and appraising the situation: The woman at the wheel is in a very bad way. He calls to the driver to bring him the oxygen bottles brought for Thaïs. Keeping his cool, the driver picks up the bottles and an emergency aid bag and runs out to join him.

I move into the back to sit next to Thaïs. She's woken up and doesn't seem to know where she is; I can see the panic in her eyes. I'm terrified too, focusing on her dilated pupils to avoid looking outside. Several painfully long minutes trickle by. I hear the emergency services arrive, lights flashing and sirens blaring. One of our ambulance men goes to meet the emergency team. He describes the situation in precise professional terms and quickly lists the care he's administered. Crucial care: a tourniquet on the woman's severed arm, oxygen, artificial respiration, keeping on talking to her. Things that save a life. Moments later, our ambulance men come back, shocked and exhausted. One of the paramedics follows them.

"Thank you for what you did," he says, "and congratulations for keeping your cool. If it weren't for you, we'd have arrived too late."

"We just did what we had to do, you know. It's just lucky we happened to be here at that exact moment with the right equipment. I think, in a way, we need to thank the little girl in this ambulance. If it weren't for her, we would never have been here."

The thrum of an air ambulance smothers the paramedic's reply. Doctors and backup teams are milling around the casualty. We're no longer needed, and we should leave to spare Thaïs the discomfort of an overly long journey. We carry on along the road without a word. Something has changed in the space of a few minutes, something that unites us in silence: a life saved because we were in the right place at the right time.

L ES VALLETS, THE PERFECT FAMILY HOME. MY PARENTS' HOME, my childhood home. With its big, boisterous happy mealtimes, its brightly colored shambles of a rumpus room, its fridge brimming with food, its blazing fires in the hearth, its cozy eiderdowns on beds that are always made up, its blackberry picking trips for making jelly, its tanning sessions beside the pool, its outings in the cart with Berthe the donkey hitched up, its tree houses, its surrounding meadows free of any habitation, its warm welcome all year round. Les Vallets, the house I love and that we all call the "happy house."

My parents are waiting impatiently for us on the doorstep. A swarm of children is looking out for us at the end of the drive; when they see the ambulance, they run toward the house, screeching, "They're here, they're here, they're coming!" The ambulance sets off along the shady drive, I catch a glimpse of the house through the leaves, and I cry with tension and relief and joy.

My parents have transformed a downstairs room into a bedroom for Thaïs—a beautiful well-lit room, which is both quiet and central, so she doesn't feel left out of family life. All the medical equipment is there and already operational, laid out in exactly the same way as in Paris for Thaïs to get her bearings. The oxygen machine to the left of the bed, the one for feeding to the right, next to the little table where we keep her medication. Every detail in place. We settle Thaïs on her bed with infinite care, and she doesn't even grimace this time, barely opening an eye and going straight back to sleep. It has to be said it's been a pretty emotional day. Everyone tiptoes out of her room, and I close the door and give an involuntary sigh. Phew, we did it. She's here and we're here, for a month.

The bags that need unpacking can wait. Barely half an hour after we arrive, two nurses come knocking at the door laden with equipment. They introduce themselves, smiling warmly: Chantal and Odile. They've come to meet their new little patient because they're going to be taking care of Thaïs while we're here.

"Exactly like the in-home care team in Paris," Chantal tells us, "well, almost exactly."

They are part of a palliative care team. I should be pleased to see them, but my throat constricts as I watch them unloading the equipment into a corner of the room and going over to Thaïs together.

Palliative care ... the expression makes me shudder. It has the same sad ring to it as a swan's song, because it so flagrantly implies that death is looming. I know Thaïs is going to die soon, but this reality is painful; and I'm balking at the thought of letting a palliative care team look after her. The nurses are familiar with this reticence from parents, so they explain what they do, taking their time, using words such as "gentle," "comfort," "pleasure," and "well-being." At no point do they define their charge in terms of the illness; they don't talk about a "patient" but a "person." Their attitude can be summarized in one sentence, "Adding life to the days when you can't add days to the life ..." That's the definition of palliative care, isn't it? It's my theme. So let's get on with it!

Chantal was right to point out that there's a difference between what they do and what the in-home care team do. She and Odile know how to stray from the beaten track of conventional medicine in order to make Thaïs's life easier. Their experience is enriched by a myriad techniques, massages, and empirical knacks. They use creams, essential oils, and ointments to give their little patient relief, with one directive: to limit the amount of medication given and simplify intervention as far as possible because treatments are more efficient the easier they are to administer. On the other hand, they're quick to use extreme measures when circumstances require—like in mid-August when Thaïs's neuropathic pain reaches a new level. With the doctor's authorization, the two nurses set up the morphine pump that the in-home care team haven't wanted to use want to use for fear that it would prove too complex or too much of a responsibility for us. Chantal and Odile don't shy away from it; they know from experience that at this stage the only way to relieve Thaïs's pain is to give her morphine continuously. They also know that we can handle the equipment because we're working toward the same goal.

Thérèse comes to join us at Les Vallets, is greeted with all these changes, and immediately adopts this innovative approach to Thaïs's care. She has no trouble getting used to it; it's how she's been doing things anyway, instinctively, for nearly a year.

Later, when we go home to Paris, we share these wonderful experiences with the in-home care nurses. They extend their care plans to include practices we learned from the palliative care team. Of course they apply them to Thaïs, but not to her alone. Plenty of sick children are still benefiting from them now.

It's fascinating. Wherever Thaïs is, children are drawn to her. In Paris, Gaspard's friends always visit her when they come to our apartment, completely naturally. We just have to take the time to explain things to them before they see her. Even so, one of them did admit as he went into the room that it gave him goose bumps . . . and there's nothing strange about that. But once by her side, not one child backs away or is put off by how she looks. Far from it, they behave remarkably normally. They're not embarrassed to inspect all the medical equipment, asking how the feeding machine works and wanting to know about the illness. They stroke her, talk to her, and play with her. Lots of them tell her she's lucky not to be at school. Childhood innocence is a wonderful thing. . . .

Thaïs has become a mascot at Les Vallets. Young and old, her cousins are happy to be spending a vacation with her and getting to know her better, and they never miss an opportunity to prove this. We haven't established any rules or imposed any limitations on visitors. We've told them that Thaïs's door is always open to them, except during her treatments. That's the only restriction, and they respect it, without fail. So, when she's not being tended to, the other children see her to their heart's content. In the morning before charging at the breakfast table, they each go to say hello to Thaïs; and in the evening, they always drop in to say goodnight. Throughout the day, they come and pay her regular little visits.

It's a universal fact: All children play, whatever their circumstances. It's a drive that goes beyond difficulties, ignores conflicts, and erases differences. Thaïs's many cousins make no departure from the rule. And they're careful to include Thaïs in their games because they're well aware that she wants to play just like them. Her illness doesn't change that. One day the gang of cousins arrange a party in Thaïs's room, with music, but not too loud, savory snacks, sodas, and great choreography. Even we, the parents, get up and dance, infected by their joy and enthusiasm.

The children don't just play with Thaïs, they're conscious of her delicate state of health and what's going to happen to her soon, and they watch out for her. They constantly come and check if she's okay and has everything she needs. Over the month of August, two lovely illustrations of this attentiveness stick in my mind and fill me with emotion.

"What are you doing here? It's very late; you should be in bed."

"I'm reading Thaïs a story so she goes to sleep and has nice dreams. It's a story about a princess."

I smile, amused and touched. With the full weight of his recently celebrated status as a four-year-old, Alex can't actually read. And he loathes tales full of princesses. And to top it all, Thaïs has already been asleep for hours. But I don't say any of that. Of course not. I reply as seriously as I can: "That's very kind of you. It's a good idea. Go on, finish the book and then get to bed quickly."

Alex carries on with his "reading," out loud and very intelligibly, concentrating hard on the thread of the story.

Jean is standing by the bed, motionless as a guardsman at Buckingham Palace; he's armed with a yellow plastic flyswatter. Before I ask any sort of question, he justifies being there: "Thaïs can't defend herself against insects that attack her, so I'm mounting the guard. As soon as I see one coming over, bang!" he explains earnestly, giving a determined whack of the flyswatter. "If the fly settles on Thaïs, I don't swat it obviously. I shoo it away with my hand, and once it's flown away, I track it down."

Jean describes his strategies without taking his eyes off a small mosquito buzzing over the bed unaware of the risk it's taking.

Thank you, children.

"When did he leave you?"
"Just over two months ago."
"Two *months*? Why did he go?"
"Another woman."

I HANG UP, SHAKEN BY WHAT I'VE JUST HEARD. DOUBLY SHAKEN: sad for this very dear friend who's been abandoned by the love of her life, and sad because she waited two long months before telling me. We used to tell each other everything, straightaway. Now, it's all different. . . .

I've spoken to her on the phone over the last couple of months, and she never said anything. Not a word, not even a hint. That silence must have taken a great deal of self-control. I can picture her holding back her tears, disguising the dull tone of her voice, clinging to pointless details to keep what mattered quiet. So much effort . . .

I know what motivated her silence. A sort of embarrassment, it's the same for everyone. "I didn't feel I could talk to you about it. It's nothing compared to what you're going through." I close my ears and my mind to it every time. Do we always have to compare our misfortunes? View them according to a hierarchy, a classification system? It's terrible to have a feeling of inferiority in your distress. If people use that line of reasoning, we'll soon be relegated to the realms of Untouchables, among those whose pain is pretty close to the top of the pyramid. Unreachable. Isolated. Despairing.

Compassion opens hearts. Mine would end up shrunken and gnarled if it didn't share the sorrows of those I love. And their joys too, of course. My, it's tough handling the guilt that happy people feel! Why does laughter die down when we come near? Why do smiles fade, faces drain of color, and fingers fidget? It's not as if I wear my distress for all to see, pinned to my chest and visible at twenty paces like a cheerleader's rosette on election night. I don't exhibit it or thrust it on people.

I want to take pleasure in good news, even the most trifling. I'd so love it if my friends carried on giving me details of their love lives, their career choices, the latest clothes they bought. I'm still interested in all that. It's not such a big part of *my* daily life, true, but it is of theirs, so I'm interested in it. I'm convinced that if you keep these conversations going, if you talk about everything and anything, then you find it easier to tackle thorny subjects. If I can laugh with them, they'll be able to cry with me because we'll still have the connection. If not, we'll grow apart until we no longer know each other.

If ever someone close to us asks me how he should behave toward us, reaching out his empty hands, palms uppermost in a gesture of impotence, I won't hesitate for a moment: "Just like before. Like everyone else. Normally."

This August evening is the night for shooting stars. The sky is the stage for a fairytale ballet. I scan the heavens, prepared to spend all evening lying unblinking on the dry grass, in the hopes of seeing a shooting star flit by, because I have something to say to it. I've only just got comfortable when I catch one; I hang on to the very end of its golden trail for a fraction of a second, just long enough to whisper my wish, "I want to carry on being Mrs. Anybody."

ONE FOOT IN FRONT OF THE OTHER. SLIGHTLY TENTATIVE. One step, then two. Rather wobbly ones. Azylis is walking! Not altogether on her own, she's holding onto Loïc's finger, but that bit of help doesn't really count, it's just to give her confidence. The main thing is she's moving forward upright on her legs, even though a bit shakily. Yes, she's walking. She's looked ready to launch herself for a few days now, but she still wasn't sure. Today she's taken the leap. She's keeping her eyes on the nearby sofa, the final destination for this adventurous epic. She takes one step after another, still holding her daddy's hand. I'm there watching, my eyes pinned on the tips of her shoes, my heart pounding.

Does her foot turn outwards? I can't help thinking about it and being afraid. I so dread suddenly spotting the imprint of the illness on Azylis in some perfectly ordinary gesture. What I fear most in the world is shakiness in her hands or a slight twist of her heel—indisputable signs of the problem afflicting her. Despite my determination to have faith, my anxiety is growing with the passing months because every day brings us closer to the critical period when visible symptoms of leukodystrophy could appear.

So, almost unconsciously, I spend my time dissecting Azylis's every move: I watch her when she drinks, when she eats, when she sits down, when she goes to bed, when she walks, when she cries. I compulsively analyze how she tackles each milestone in life, trying to remember how Gaspard did it. And particularly how Thaïs did . . .

Does her foot turn outwards, then? It doesn't seem to, not at first sight. No, I don't think it does. Unless I'm not looking closely enough. But my eyes are stinging—I'm staring so hard at the ends of her shoes. I can't work out what I'm seeing anymore. I haven't even enjoyed my baby daughter's first steps; I haven't even acknowledged her achievement. I've let this uncontrollable terror overrun me. I sit on the sofa she's just reached with such glory, as others might reach the summit of Mont Blanc, and I cry. Tears of fear mingled with tears of pride. I congratulate Azylis by hugging her to me, a little too hard.

"Well done, my darling, you're walking!"

Yes, she's walking. But Thaïs used to walk too. And yet . . .

We haven't noticed the time passing. That's how you know you're enjoying yourself. The month of August has sped by: I feel as if we arrived yesterday and we already need to pack up our bags, tidy the house, and head back the way we came. The cousins part with promises to meet up again soon. The goodbyes are tearful; no one likes vacations coming to an end.

The ambulance men, the same ones, are punctual, and the return journey isn't as stressful as the outbound one: A few hours later, the ambulance arrives at our destination without incident. We're back home once more, and we quickly get back into our routine.

Thaïs is happy to be with her beloved nurses and physical therapist again. They're happy to see her too after this month-long separation. Despite their joy, I can tell they've noticed changes in their patient. We ourselves are aware her condition has altered.

All through August we had no major fears, like the one in the spring or last Christmas, but a host of little anxieties: With no obvious reason why, her heart-rate would speed up or slow down, her breathing would stop for a while or her temperature take off. Every incident is dangerous, and Thaïs never comes out of them completely unharmed. She spends most of her time dozing, and sadly not only because of the morphine. This lethargy is becoming more and more like a loss of consciousness. Leukodystrophy is making its mark deep down now, right into the connections in Thaïs's brain.

These periods of light coma give me a peculiar feeling. Thaïs may well look as if she's sleeping serenely, but you can tell this is no ordinary sleep. At times like this, she emanates a particular sort of density. The intensity of her unconscious presence is so powerful that it makes us talk to her and treat her as if she were awake.

I always feel incredibly relieved when Thaïs emerges from these sluggish periods, because I'm always afraid she won't come back. The doctors predicted that her death was imminent in December, but despite expectations, Thaïs is still here nine months later. Gaspard is actually convinced his sister's immortal.

Children with leukodystrophy often die of the effects of a respiratory problem or of a chronic infection. Thaïs hasn't had this sort of complication since Christmas; she hasn't caught the slightest virus or the tiniest bug. I'm utterly convinced that Thaïs is going to go all the way with this illness. And I feel that the end is striding ever closer.

Tomorrow is back-to-school day. Gaspard has everything ready; he's sharpened his pencils, sorted out his books, folded his overall. A buckled satchel is sitting in pride of place in the hallway, ready for the big day. Just one satchel. Thaïs won't be going to school tomorrow. Not tomorrow, not ever.

Tomorrow, every child her age will head off to nursery school, walking bravely, accompanied by proud, emotional, stressed-out parents. Tomorrow, Thaïs's day will be like today, and the day before, and the day before that. She won't get up, won't get dressed, won't put her satchel on her back, won't squeeze my hand when she steps into a classroom for the first time. Tomorrow nothing special will happen for her; she'll follow the usual succession of nurses, physical therapist, and the man delivering gas bottles and food pouches. Her own routine.

Tomorrow, on his way to school, Gaspard will keep his head lowered, sad that Thaïs isn't going to school like him. I'll hear him mumbling under his breath, working out which grade he will be in when Azylis comes to school; crossing his fingers in the hope he'll still be in elementary school with her. I won't dare tell him that she may never be up to going to school. I'll say nothing because I have no idea about Azylis's future. I'll leave his hopes intact.

Tomorrow, Gaspard will cry in my arms, for a long time, outside the door to his new school—like lots of other kids perhaps, but not for the same reasons. He'll cry, devastated that he's the only child in his family to go to school. As I console him, I'll gauge what a heavy burden normality can be to bear when it becomes the exception.

Tomorrow, before going into school, Gaspard will formulate one last request through clenched jaws: "Mommy, could you explain to my class about Thaïs? And about Azylis too? Please. I'd prefer it if you did it. It'll be better. The kids'll believe you."

Tomorrow, our mountain will feel like the Himalayas. Only bigger.

W E'RE TURNING A NEW PAGE. AND NOT JUST ANY PAGE. A great big one, written with a tremulous hand: the transplant page. A year after the operation, it's all over. Azylis has an ordinary immune system and plenty of blood cells. Everything's back to normal, and Azylis no longer needs to go to the hospital for transplant follow-up tests. She'll just have a blood test from time to time and an annual checkup. Not much more than that, at least as far as the transplant is concerned. As for monitoring the illness, things haven't changed: Azylis will continue to have tests every three months to check how the situation is evolving, and we don't know when those appointments will stop. If they ever do.

Right now, we've turned the transplant page once and for all. It's crazy, but as the months passed by, I eventually forgot this stage would come to an end. Something transitory had taken root in our lives. I grew accustomed to the regular trips to and from the hospital; they'd become a routine part of our lives. As I turn the page, I realize I have absolutely no regrets or remorse about this period; I don't even have bad memories of it. Perhaps memory is selective and retains only the best moments so we can tolerate the past. I'll just remember a general feeling of tiredness at various points, a few unpleasant impressions, such as my terror on the day of the transplant itself or how frightened we were when the doctors deliberately provoked a graft versus host response. But nothing serious. No wound. No scar.

This page takes another one in its wake, one that follows the trend and turns over too. This is a page I've hated: Azylis's medication. For months we had a daily struggle to get her to swallow wretched tablets and horrible syrups. Every day, we battled against her retching and ignored her tears, telling ourselves over and over that it was for her good. Every time I cursed as I wondered, *Why?* Why don't the pharmaceuticals labs make drugs that are practical for children?

As soon as you venture away from the classic strawberry-flavored syrups for fevers and mild pain relief, children's medication becomes a real headache. Drugs aren't of suitable form or taste for the very young. They're acrid, bitter, rasping, cloying, grainy, disgusting. They come in the form of capsules or tablets, which are impossible for children to swallow. We always had to open the capsules or crush the tablets, dissolve them in water, and then get our recalcitrant daughter to drink them, praying she wouldn't spit it all out. More than once I thought longingly of Thaïs's gastrostomy, which facilitated the administration of all her medication.

These constraining rituals are behind us now, and that makes me happy—for our sakes, but more importantly for Azylis's. Her life is more and more like the one other little girls her age lead.

It always amazes me: Every time someone goes into Thaïs's room and she's not asleep, she turns her head toward the visitor. And when someone comes over to the bed, she very obviously turns to face the person, whichever side of the bed he or she stands on. How does Thaïs know so accurately whereabouts in the room we are? It's a real mystery.

Today, still, she welcomes me by stretching her neck toward me. I go right over to her and start talking to her gently as I lean over her.

Just then she turns her head away from me, where there's no one. I walk around the bed to get back into her "line of sight." She turns the other way again. What's going on? Is she angry? She doesn't *look* upset. I move again; her head swivels in the opposite direction.

After several fruitless attempts, I start worrying. Has Thaïs lost the instinctive compass that makes her always turns toward us? Has she now been deprived of this sixth sense which means she can sense us without seeing or hearing us? It's only then that I hear a little purring sound that we all recognize: Thaïs is laughing!

Everything becomes clear. Thanks to her laughter, I realize she's actually playing a trick on me. She's playing hide-and-seek, that's all. It's always been her favorite game, so she's found a way to carry on playing it. A child's imagination has no limits. Like babies who think they disappear when they hide behind their hands, Thaïs thinks she's invisible just by turning her head the other way.

I'm eternally grateful for this magic moment when a little girl imperiously thumbed her nose at her illness. Nothing can stop her playing. Like the boy with his electric train.

Won over by her irresistible ingenuousness, I throw myself into her game, pretending I can't find her. Relying heavily on gestures and sounds, I search frantically for her as if I can't see her, even though she's right in the middle of the room—and the very heart of my life.

THE EASEL IS SET UP, THE BRUSHES READY, THE PALETTE prepared. The talented Bertrand sets to work. Painting Thaïs is his idea, immortalizing her as she is today: beautiful, so beautiful.

Our friend Bertrand has enough talent, experience, and ability to save him from the terrors of a blank canvas, but it's a long time before he applies the first touch with his brush. He knows everything this portrait will mean to us later, when Thaïs is gone. Photos are sometimes crude because they can't disguise any of the reality. Painting is more tactful. It can smudge out unsightly tubes and erase imposing machines, keeping only what really matters: a pretty little girl asleep on her bed.

Alone with her, he absorbs the feel of the room, of Thaïs's favorite treasures, her world, everything that describes her and so aptly represents who she is. Then, driven by a creative urge, he applies himself to the job. Thaïs isn't a difficult subject to paint, she's not impatient, doesn't throw tantrums or suffer from cramps. She holds her pose effortlessly, in fact she doesn't move a muscle because she's sound asleep. In the sort of sleep that is now so common, hovering on the edge of unconsciousness.

A few hours later the artist is putting the finishing touches to his painting. And then, as if aware her visitor's about to leave, Thaïs wakes up. She barely opens one eye, but it's enough to reveal a little glow of life. With his eyes pinned on his model, Bertrand takes up his brushes again, and in two or three expert flourishes he transforms his work. In the gap between her eyelids he puts a shining pinpoint of black. He draws out the corners of her lips and tints them a stronger red. These small details reveal Thaïs's smile and light up the picture.

Ah, Thaïs's smile! It would make the Mona Lisa pale with jealousy. An inimitable smile, a gentle combination of innocence and maturity, of joy and seriousness. A smile that's never feigned and comes from so far away, from the depths of her beautiful soul. It sneaks into the sparkle of her eyes, under her long eyelashes and into the subtle movement of her mouth. This isn't the sort of smile that shows her teeth—Thaïs can't do that; her features aren't mobile enough. No, it's the sort that shows her heart.

No present has ever felt so precious to us as this lovely painting. Bertrand didn't settle for just capturing Thaïs's face in a pretty picture: Beneath the still gleaming varnish, he's captured forever her personality, her essence, her spirit, her life. And her smile.

Three and three-quarter years. Today Thaïs is exactly three and three-quarter years old. She's so young: so young we're still counting the quarters. For her, this year that's passed so densely and intensely should count as double. She's so nearly four she can almost touch it. Just three more months. Or rather, a whole three months to go! Will she have the strength to get there? Her birthday feels like a mirage in the desert that gets further away the closer we get to it. The days separating us from that date are going by too slowly. But I'm hanging on because I want to celebrate this birthday with her. This one more than any other: It's a leap year, with a precious February 29. On that day she will unquestionably be four years old.

Thaïs has had only one normal birthday in her life: her first. We celebrated it in a happy carefree way. We didn't know. . . . The day she turned two will always be engraved on our hearts as one of the darkest of our lives. When she was three, we made use of the situation. When someone's born on February 29, you can decide whether you celebrate their birthday on February 28 or March 1; it seemed logical to us always to celebrate it the day after February 28. Anyway, the year she was three, we bent the rule: we celebrated it on February 28 and March 1. Two happy days instead of one. One way of finding some consolation. Seeing as she won't live for long, we doubled up her birthday, without aging her any more quickly.

Everything's different this year: The calendar has a February 29. I'm clinging to that day, praying Thaïs will still be with us then.

Several bereaved mothers have told me that their children's birthdays are more difficult to cope with than the anniversaries of their deaths. I feel the same. Every year, memories of that day come back to me, intact. I remember the sweet elation, the boundless emotion, the promise of life hugged close to me. All the plans, the hopes, the future with that tiny newborn.

I have painfully lucid memories of the enormous happiness I felt when Thaïs came into the world. When I found out she was a girl, I could have burst with joy. A girl, a princess ... I'd been longing for one. While the midwife checked her over, I smiled beatifically as I pictured everything I would do with her. I saw her as a five-year-old twirling in pretty dresses, as a fifteen-year-old going to great lengths to look gorgeous, as a twenty-year-old, already a woman. I liked everything I saw. I anticipated our mother-daughter complicity. And I felt strong. Thaïs was giving me a sense of balance, of trust in life. Perhaps that trust was a little naïve, but it was so sincere. I thought that now, whatever happened, I had a daughter. Whatever happened ...

For a long time, I regretted that Thaïs was born on February 29. Now, I'm convinced it's better that way. I tell myself I'll have to relive the day she was born only once every four years. The other years I'll take refuge in vagaries of the calendar. I'll sidle off between February 28 and March 1, to cry, where no one can see me.

The results have merely confirmed what we already knew. Azylis is going downhill. In two months her walking hasn't improved, she's never let go of her father's finger. Every valiant attempt to launch out on her own ended in a fall. This lack of progress in itself was a bad sign. Until I saw it very clearly: Her feet now turn outwards. Not entirely in the same way as Thaïs's, but they turn all the same. And they slow her down. And her hands shake. Not all the time, only sometimes, when she brings a spoon to her mouth or reaches out her hand. The evidence is staring me in the face: The illness is developing in Azylis.

The truth feels even more brutal when I read it in her medical report. This month's tests disguise nothing: Her nerve conductivity is slowing in the peripheral nervous system, and her motor faculties are deteriorating. These developments aren't under control. Yes, that's right, Azylis is falling back. And I'm falling apart.

I've lost my strength, my voice, the light in my eyes. This situation is a cruel reenactment of eighteen months ago, when we heard the name metachromatic leukodystrophy for the first time.

The doctor isn't ready to admit defeat. In his view, the news is bad of course, but there's nothing catastrophic about it. Deterioration of the peripheral nervous system was predictable because the illness was developing all through the year that it took for the transplant to have effect. It was a close-run race, perhaps an unwinnable one. But these aren't the only results. Others are more encouraging. He begs me to focus on the positive things: Azylis's MRI scan is still perfect; there are no detectable alterations in her brain, and all the psycho-motor tests are normal. That certainly wouldn't have been the case without the transplant. It's had a beneficial effect on Azylis, that's for sure. All hope is not lost: The changes in her motor functions could stabilize at a later date.

It's all the same to me because I don't believe in it anymore. Azylis will never get better, at least not completely. In a few weeks, a few months at the outside, she'll lose the ability to walk, then to stand, then to sit, then to speak, then everything else, since no one can stop this godforsaken illness.

I don't feel rebellious or angry. Just terribly weak, hugely discouraged, and profoundly weary. And, of course, I can still hear them, those words, still the same ones, the ever present "if you knew." But that's just it: I don't know. And I'm tired of all this uncertainty.

Whatever the night is like, the sun comes up. It will take time for me to climb back up the hill and find renewed hope, but I'll get there. With Loïc. One step at a time.

When we read the results of those tests yesterday, we weren't hearing for the first time that Azylis was ill; we've known that since her birth. Since then we've battled on and never backed down. And, tiny and fragile as she was, she fought hard too. Without giving up. A struggle she's undertaken in her own way, with no other weapons than her love of life, her boundless energy, her sunny nature ... and her trust. She too can tell that her situation is getting more complicated. She's well aware that her body no longer obeys her in quite the same way, but she's still not faltering. This morning, like yesterday, she picked up her weapons and set out once more to conquer life, taking us along with her.

Darling little Azylis, I have no idea what your life will be like. I don't know whether you'll go down the same road as Thaïs, or join Gaspard on his, or whether you'll map one out just for you. But we'll be on that road with you, every day. And if you can't walk, we'll carry you to make sure you get further along the way.

Darling little Azylis, we believe in you, we have faith in you. We won't abandon you. Not today or ever. In this war we're waging but over which we have no control, the greatest support we can offer you is our love. Our unconditional love.

Yes, my darling little Azylis, it's you that I love, not your abilities and aptitudes. It's you, for who you are. Not for what you do.

For your whole life, my darling little Azylis.

ONE NIGHT. IF THERE HAD TO BE JUST ONE NIGHT, IT WOULD be this one—this cold, dark December night. It starts like every other, with my trying to find elusive sleep, struggling with turbulent dreams. And yet this night was to change my life. Forever.

Three o'clock in the morning. A time when all certainties waver, snared in the suddenly hostile depths of a darkness grown too black. The previous day seems far away. The next dawn is still hesitating to break. I'm not asleep, despite my heavy eyelids. My mind goes over and over things; my heart rate quickens. I have to go to her. As I do on so many nights.

I get up softly and walk through the sleeping apartment, annoyed with the old wooden floor for creaking underfoot. I don't want to wake anyone, don't want any witnesses to my nocturnal escapade. I go into Thaïs's bedroom but don't turn on the light; I don't need it. The machines purr to a soothing rhythm. Her oxygen level appears as a luminous red dot. Thaïs is lying on her bed, motionless as usual, her head turned toward the door and her eyes closed. She's sleeping peacefully. I draw up a chair to sit beside her, and take her warm chubby hand. Shrouded in silence, I gaze at her. Not moving or talking, I just stay there, and the night draws itself out gently.

As they grow used to the dark, my eyes make out the room: the machines and sensors, the cuddly toys and dolls, the embroidered sheet, the children's drawings pinned to the wall. I'm filled with emotion as I look around Thaïs's world. When my eyes come to rest on her, they meet hers. I thought she was asleep, but her eyes are staring up at me, wide open. Their sudden intensity is uncomfortable. Thaïs can't see now, and all at once this blind stare of hers cuts right through me, delving its way right to my heart.

It takes courage on my part to hold her gaze—and surrender to it. Time stands still. I can't even be sure my heart's still beating. Nothing exists now except for those ebony eyes. There in the depths of a winter's night—my attention pinned on my daughter's eyes, her hand held tightly in mine—our hearts and minds and souls are in communion, and I understand. At last.

It feels like a blinding explosion. Without moving or speaking, Thaïs reveals a secret, the most beautiful and longed for secret: Love. With a capital letter.

One day, in a hospital consulting room, I promised my sick little girl that I would pass on to her everything I knew about this emotion that makes the world go round. I've made a point of doing that for eighteen months. And all that time, too absorbed by the sheer scale of the task, I didn't see, I didn't grasp that she was the one teaching me about love. In all those months spent by her side, I didn't realize because actually, when I come to think of it, I don't know much about love, real love.

How does she know? How is it possible? Thaïs has been deprived of everything. She can't move, can't talk, can't hear, can't sing, can't laugh, and can't see. She can't even cry. But she loves. That's all she does, with all her strength. Through her wounds and infirmities and failings.

Thaïs's love doesn't impose itself, it exposes itself, reveals itself. She appears to us as she is, fragile and vulnerable, with no shell or armor or shields. With no fear. Of course someone looking from a distance can scoff at, scorn, or spurn this fragile state. But all who come nearer, who lean in close and try to follow her journey, they like me will see that this vulnerability elicits only one response: love.

Almost two years ago, hearing the extent of the damage this illness would cause, I asked myself something, "What will she have left?" Love. She will be left with love. The love we receive. And the love we give too.

Yes, love has the unique ability to reverse the current, to change weakness into strength. Deprived of her senses and physically dependent, Thaïs can't really do anything without outside assistance. She could ask a lot, and yet all she expects from us is what we willingly give her. Nothing more.

We generally think that a painful, diminished life is hard to accept, and that's probably true if you don't have love. What's unbearable is the absence of love. When you love and are loved in return, you can cope with everything. Even pain. Even suffering. Suffering ... we know so much about it, this unwelcome companion to our lives, and we've experienced it in all its guises. All except one perhaps: the one that nudges people toward despair, that annihilates the best of feelings. Yes, I realize tonight that I've never suffered because of Thaïs. Never. I've suffered *with* her a great deal, far too much, all the time. But always together.

This evening I'll venture to say it: Thaïs's life is a treasure, a concentrate of love that she generously diffuses around her. How many people have come to visit her, out of solidarity or compassion or affection, it doesn't really matter why, and then left bowled over, turned upside down. But not bowled over in the sense of confronting a brutal shock, not destroyed, not traumatized. No, bowled over because they saw something else, beyond the pain and physical weakness. They glimpsed a far more contagious illness. . . .

I remember one of the night nurses in Marseille. I didn't hear her come into Thaïs's room, and she stayed there a while, busying around my daughter, but didn't go straight back out afterwards. She sat down on the end of my bed and confided in a husky voice: "What's going on here? There's something special in this room. I don't know what it is, but it's unique. You're up against the worst, and yet you feel good. There's such a sense of gentleness, happiness even. Sorry if what I'm saying upsets you, but I can't keep it to myself." At the time I didn't grasp what she meant. Now, it's all become clear.

Without looking away from her penetrating stare, I move closer still to Thaïs, until my face brushes against hers, and gazing into her eyes, I whisper: "Thank you, Thaïs. For everything. For who you are. Everything you are. And for everything you give. You make us so happy. Really happy. I love you, my princess."

Deep in the heart of me, the voice fades away and leaves me alone. My mind has stopped ringing with that never ending "If you knew ..." My heart explodes with a cry, "I know!"

A SIGH. JUST ONE. LONG AND DEEP. IT REVERBERATES powerfully through the silence of this night before Christmas.

Leaning close in beside our daughter, Loïc and I hold our breath to gather in hers. The last. Thaïs has just died.

Good-bye now, my little Thaïs.

ACKNOWLEDGEMENTS

To my parents and parents-in-law, thank you for the time, energy, and love that you've given us without counting the cost.

To Thérèse, thank you for your joyfulness, your soothing presence, your reassuring reliability, and all the wonderful things you brought to our family.

To the frontline troops: Zabeth, Caro, Solène, Béné, Louis-Étienne, Malex, Marie-Pascale, Arlette, and Anne-Marie; to the invincible: Constance, Antoine, Sophie, Damien, Nico, and Bertrand; thank you for never giving up.

To the members of the in-home care team: Delphine, Bénédicte, Laure, Delphine, and Édith G.; to the palliative care nurses: Odile and Chantal; to the doctors, Patrick A. and Caroline S. along with their team, particularly Christine, Florence, Adèle, and Marie-Claude B., an astute psychologist; to the physical therapist Jérôme G.; to the UPIX team; thank you for your skill, for being there with us and having faith in us.

To EAL, thank you for helping us climb our mountains.

To Chantal, Laurence, and their family, thank you for your generosity and for such a warm welcome.

To my sisters, Marie-Edmée and Amicie, thank you for being there, in the bad times but also in the good.

To Father François, thank you for showing us—so often—that we shouldn't lose sight of what really matters.

To Christian, thank you for pushing me to go that step further.

Lastly, to Loïc, thank you—for everything.

And thank you to all those who have supported us by being there and keeping us in their thoughts or prayers. And still do.